RECENT CONTRIBUTIONS TO NEUROPHYSIOLOGY

RECENT CONTRIBUTIONS TO NEUROPHYSIOLOGY

International Symposium in Neurosciences in Honor
of Herbert H. Jasper

Colloque International en Sciences Neurologiques en Hommage
à Herbert H. Jasper

EDITED BY

JEAN-PIERRE CORDEAU

Université de Montréal, Montréal (Canada)

AND

PIERRE GLOOR

McGill University, Montreal (Canada)

ELECTROENCEPHALOGRAPHY AND CLINICAL
NEUROPHYSIOLOGY
SUPPLEMENT NO. 31

ELSEVIER PUBLISHING COMPANY
AMSTERDAM/LONDON/NEW YORK

Electroenceph. clin. Neurophysiol., **1972**, *Suppl. 31*

ELSEVIER PUBLISHING COMPANY
335 JAN VAN GALENSTRAAT
P.O. BOX 211, AMSTERDAM, THE NETHERLANDS

AMERICAN ELSEVIER PUBLISHING COMPANY, INC.
52 VANDERBILT AVENUE
NEW YORK, NEW YORK 10017

Library of Congress Card Number: 72–83205
ISBN 0–444–40963–7
With 123 illustrations and 10 tables.

Printed in the Netherlands.

Contents

Editor's note

While this volume was in preparation for publication my co-editor, Dr. Jean-Pierre Cordeau, unexpectedly died. I lost not only a co-worker, but also a dear friend with whom it was a delight to collaborate both in editing this book and, during the preceding year, in planning and preparing the meeting in honor of Dr. Herbert H. Jasper at which the papers published in this volume were presented. The success of this meeting was largely due to Jean-Pierre Cordeau's initiative and dedication. Without him the symposium would not have been what it was, a heart warming reunion of friends and an exciting scientific meeting. Jean-Pierre Cordeau's death left a great void among his friends and collaborators. None of us who worked with him on this project suspected that this book would be his last publication.

Montreal, 5 November 1971.   P. GLOOR, M. D.

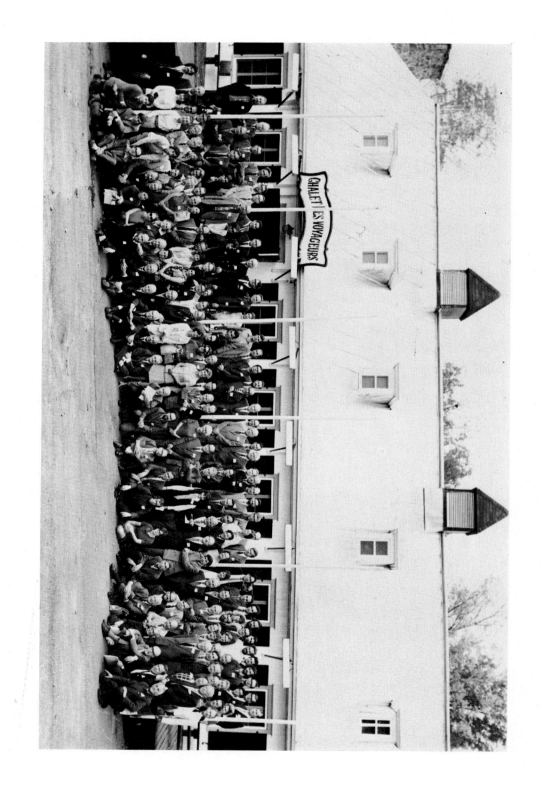

Foreword

Over the past three decades we have witnessed an astonishing growth of the neurosciences which has greatly advanced our understanding of the noblest organ of man, his brain. Many pioneers have contributed to make this science of the brain the exciting and promising topic it is today. This volume is dedicated to honor one of those pioneers, Dr. Herbert H. Jasper, who perhaps more than anyone else has realized that in order to truly serve the study of man and his brain, basic neurological sciences must walk hand in hand with their clinical sister disciplines in a true mutual partnership. Basic science must create the foundation upon which clinical knowledge and treatment should rest; the clinical sciences must pose to the basic scientists the relevant and provocative questions which need to be answered if we wish to further our understanding of the mysteries enshrined in the human brain.

In the early autumn of 1970, from the 24th to the 26th of September, more than two hundred former students, co-workers and friends of Dr. Herbert H. Jasper congregated at Mont Tremblant in the Laurentian mountains north of Montreal to pay tribute to the man who had inspired their work and to whom they owe much of their own dedication to the study of brain sciences. The hardwood forest of the Laurentian shield had put on for the occasion its glorious autumn finery in a riotous outburst of colours. Neuroscientists came from many parts of the world. Some came bearing gifts in the form of scientific papers which were presented during these memorable three days, many more came to listen and, by their presence, to pay homage to a beloved fellow scientist, teacher and friend. The organizers of the symposium felt that the opportunity should not be missed to make accesssible to a wider public the rich scientific lore presented at this meeting. This volume thus constitutes a collection of the papers read at this symposium. They cover a wide spectrum, ranging from basic fundamental biophysics through sophisticated microneurophysiology all the way to clinical electroencephalography and clinical neurology. The variety of topics reflects the breadth of Dr. Jasper's own far-ranging scientific interests. This volume also contains, in lieu of a preface, two very personal contributions. They are the texts of two after-dinner speeches, one presented by Lord Adrian and the other by Dr. Wilder Penfield. Both pay homage to Herbert Jasper, the man and the scientist. They reflect the personal warmth of affection towards him which found so vivid and tangible an expression during these three memorable days.

Montreal, February 1971   P. GLOOR and J. P. CORDEAU

Forty Years' Progress in Neurophysiology

We have come to celebrate Herbert Jasper's career and to thank him for all he has done for the science of neurophysiology both by his own researches and by giving so much of his time in helping to establish the subdivision of clinical electroencephalography, to make it a going concern, with a journal of its own and an international congress.

I was asked to speak about the progress of neurophysiology in the last 40 years, and I will try to do so, though I have forgotten a good deal that happened between 1930 and 1950 and have failed to assimilate all the advances which have been made between 1950 and 1970. But I do remember the time when Jasper started his career as a neurophysiologist in 1931. He was then an instructor at the University of Iowa, but he was given a National Research Council Fellowship to work in physiology, at the University of Paris and in the department of Professor Lapicque and I read several papers he published with Professor A. M. Monnier. I know very little about his earlier work in psychology but you may be interested in the title of Jasper's first scientific paper. It was published in 1930 in the *American Journal of Sociology* and the title has a modern ring: it was "Optimism and Pessimism in College Environment". Perhaps if Herbert had stuck to psychology we should know better how to deal with campus unrest, though we should be that much less able to use the electroencephalograph as an aid to its diagnosis. But I have mentioned Herbert Jasper's start in psychology for it shows, perhaps, how his interests are involved with the finished product—the intelligent organism—as well as with all the nerve cell systems which make it behave as it does. In 1931, however, Hans Berger's work on the electroencephalogram was largely unknown and Jasper's research in Paris was concerned with the chronaxie, Lapicque's "Time Constant for Excitation".

Now in these last 40 years there have, of course, been major advances in the science of neurophysiology apart altogether from the development of electroencephalography for clinical purposes, but in the first 10 years of the period, that is from 1930–40, I think it would be agreed that the most impressive development was in the field of the human EEG. In 1930 few of us had any knowledge of Berger's work but by 1937 it was already the centre of interest at the International Congress of Psychology in Paris. It was on this subject that Jasper began to work when he came back to the U.S.A. in 1935, and he was one of the pioneers who helped to secure its recognition as a field for research in neurophysiology and not only an aid to clinical diagnosis.

Apart from the EEG, however, in the years from 1930–40 research on the electrical activity of the brain had been somewhat disappointing, though the reason was simply the contrast from the previous decade 1920–30. Then we were learning a new technique of electrical recording which was just what was needed for research on peripheral nerves, but it was only a partial answer when it was used in the thirties for research on the cerebral cortex. In fact, the technique of triode amplification had been a godsend in work on nervous conduction and on the activity in fibres, but at first it was almost a hindrance to research on the cortical neurones. The difficulties there arose not so much from insensitive recording as from the complexity of the structures, the tangle of cells and dendrites, from which records had to be made. There was technical progress, of course, in the thirties on this and on other lines: operations on the brain became easier with the barbiturates as anaesthetics and there were Bremer's preparations of isolated parts of the brain, the *cerveau isolé* and the *encéphale isolé*. But the neuroanatomists were chiefly engaged in tracing the complex pathways below the cerebrum and soon the focus of interest of many neurophysiologists was shifting from the cerebrum to the brain stem and particularly to the reticular formation.

However, apart from electrical recordings, in the period 1930–40 there had been plenty of activity in other kinds of research on the nervous system, at various levels. In the U.S.S.R. the pupils of Pavlov were deeply engaged in their work on conditioned reflexes. In the U.S.A., there was Lashley's continued search for the engram, the substrata of learned behaviour. There were the suppressor strips on the cortical surface found by Dusser de Barenne and McCulloch and there were the observations of Fulton and Jacobsen on the frontal lobes of the chimpanzee which led Moniz to use pre-frontal leucotomy for the treatment of mental disorders. Hess had begun his work on the induction of sleep by stimulation of the thalamus, and throughout the period there was mounting evidence for the theory of transmission from nerve to muscle by chemical agents. It had been put forward and strongly supported by Dale and Loewi, but was doubted by some of the electrophysiologists.

I have mentioned only some of the highlights, but they are enough to show that neurophysiology had made some progress in 1930–40; and some of you may have noticed that in the list I have given there are the names of five Nobel prizewinners. With the financial depression everywhere and Europe distracted by threats of war and by racial hatreds, this is not a bad record for one branch of physiology. But after the war the gains have been far more substantial. We have been greatly assisted, of course, by the phenomenal progress of physical and chemical technology. In the field of brain physiology we have gone deeper with microelectrodes, wider with invertebrates and higher with mathematics. We can study the structure of cells and of molecules with the electron microscope and the X–ray spectrometer and we can separate intractable mixtures by chromatography. We have found many new problems to puzzle the rising generation and some that troubled their elders have now been comfortably settled. There was one in particular which was badly in need of solution. I have already mentioned the work of Dale and Loewi on chemical transmission from nerve fibre to muscle. In the thirties and forties it was often suggested that the signals were passed across the gap from synapse to neurone by a discharge of acetylcholine and not by the electrical change. But some form of electrical transmission could not be quite ruled out. There were ardent supporters of chemical transmission in the central nervous system, there were stubborn objectors, and some of us sat on the fence. We remained on the fence in mounting discomfort until 1950, when the point was settled with the aid of a further development which had taken place in the technique of electrical recording, the use of tubular microelectrodes to lead from within the cell. With this method Eccles produced conclusive evidence in favour of chemical (or at least non-electrical) transmission, for there was a definite iso-electrical interval when transmission from afferent synapse to motor neurone was taking place.

That was 20 years ago and since then a great deal of information has been gained on synaptic transmission: there has been no certain identification of other transmitters than acetylcholine, though several have been suggested. Recording with microelectrodes has also been used to great advantage in providing a detailed description of neural mechanics in the cerebellum as well as the brain stem. A more recent development has been the mapping of the cortical neurones which receive the sensory information. I am thinking particularly of the work of Hubel and Wiesel on the cells of the visual area of the cortex and of that of Mountcastle on those in the tactile area. In the visual area there is a columnar arrangement of neurones which are grouped into patterns of excitation and inhibition related to significant features of the sensory stimulus, the direction of movement, for instance, or the balance of light and shade. In the tactile area there is also a columnar arrangement of cortical cells and similar patterns of excitation and inhibition: with visual stimuli the analysis has already begun in the retinal layers and Hartline's studies have emphasized once again the importance of inhibition as a constant partner to excitation in regions where networks exist.

Once more I must try not to give the impression that all the advances in neurophysiology since 1950 have come from electrical records. But in the period from 1950 until today there have been so many new developments that I can only refer you to a volume of nearly 1,000 pages entitled *The Neurosciences* and published by the Rockefeller University three years ago. In it you will find accounts of the latest research on sleep, on memory and learning, on the split-brain preparation, on the molecular biology of brain cells, the storage of information by bacteria and the enhancement of learning by drugs. And if this is not enough there are countless new journals to choose from and new meetings to attend as well as the 33 volumes of the *Journal of Neurophysiology* which was started in 1938.

You will scarcely need to be told of the other journal which was started 11 years later—in 1949. Some of you may have read the volumes of the "EEG Journal" *(Electroencephalography and Clinical Neurophysiology)* from cover to cover: at all events Herbert Jasper can scarcely have avoided the task (or the pleasure) at least for the first 12 volumes. For he was its editor or editor in chief until 1962. I am coming to some of the lines of research that Jasper has followed in recent years, but I do not think research should get all the credit. As a rule the scientists who edit our journals get very little—their work is taken for granted. We regard them as worthy colleagues, unselfish enough to toil for the good of the subject and honest enough to reject the impossible papers, whoever submits them. They cannot expect to be thanked by the authors whose papers they have shortened or rewritten, but readers and even authors can be grateful when an editor like Herbert Jasper is holding the reins. He has made the journal a model to all the others which deal with new branches of science at the international level. It has guided the development of electroencephalography without letting it lose its identity or poaching on other fields: the papers are written (or edited) so that we can see what the authors have done and why they have done it. We can follow the progress in every branch of the subject and in every part of the world.

But the EEG Journal could never have been guided so well if the editor had stayed all day in his office, if he had not been one of the leaders, with experiments to be done and papers of his own to be written. In the early days he had convinced us that the alpha rhythm was not confined to the occipital region. In Cambridge we had supposed that it must be, on the basis of records from very few subjects (who happened, perhaps, to fit with our preconceptions of how the rhythm arose). But it was clear that Jasper was right. Till the end of the thirties, however, the interest chiefly arose from the clinical uses of EEG recording. Grey Walter had shown it could help in locating cerebral tumours, Gibbs, Davis and Lennox had made many records of epileptic discharges, Jasper and Andrews, and Loomis and his team had studied the rhythms in the different stages of sleep and there had been many attempts to find special features in the records from patients with neurosis or mental disorder.

In 1938 Jasper had moved from Brown to Montreal to join Wilder Penfield's team at McGill as the expert on electrical methods. It was an excellent move for the progress of electroencephalography for in 1941 Penfield and Erickson published their book on "Epilepsy and Cerebral Localisation" with a chapter of 75 pages by Herbert Jasper on the electrical evidence. It was in Penfield's Institute at McGill early in 1942 that I first saw Jasper in action, in an operating theatre which was then the last word for the use of electrical recording in cranial surgery. They were stimulating the temporal lobe and recording patients' impressions and the potentials in the cortex. I had tried to record from the human cortex myself some years earlier with portable apparatus in an unshielded theatre at the London Hospital where Cairns was the neurosurgeon, so I was lost in admiration at Jasper's technique, which ran so smoothly and gave such consistent results. But the titles of Jasper's papers during the war remind one of other medical problems, traumatic epilepsy, the effect of sulphanilamide crystals on the cortex (before penicillin arrived), EEG studies of head wounds and the rate of recovery from nerve injuries.

After the war the International EEG Organization was set up in 1947 with Jasper as President and editor of its journal as well. And since then he has been in constant demand because of his talents for organization and his knowledge of the international effort in science. One expects to see him at all the congresses on the brain or on electroencephalography, and when IBRO, the International Brain Research Organization, was started in 1961 he could not avoid the demand that he should be secretary in charge of the office in Paris.

But although he is one of our pioneers and is now an elder statesman he has never allowed himself to be separated for long from his laboratory; his output of research has rarely been interrupted. He has had many collaborators and has published a series of papers, mainly concerned with the effects of attention, learning, sleep, distraction, etc., on the electrical activity of different regions of the animal brain. His papers have set a high standard. He is fertile in trying new situations and honest in reporting results, for the observations are set out dispassionately however much is at stake.

So what is the position we have reached? It looks as though work on the brain has come to a difficult, perhaps a critical stage, but this is a sign of the right sort of progress; it is not a confession of failure now or in the future.

The electroencephalographer can lead from the scalp and recognize features in the tracings which are signs of cerebral disorder. There is probably room for improvement in technical methods and for enlarging the search for specific indications of disease which the EEG can give. When it is recorded for clinical uses, however, we need not be specially concerned at our ignorance of all but the outlines of the cerebral machinery which is producing the record. But the neurophysiologist is trying to understand much more than the outlines. His problem is how the cerebrum makes us behave as intelligent people with memories and skills and knowledge of good and evil. He must study the interactions in the elaborate structure of thousands of millions of cells which come into action when a sense organ is stimulated and the appropriate response is given.

We can lead from the surface of the brain to record the cortical waves or we can lead from the cells with microelectrodes to record the unit activity, but there is not much relation between them. When we try to relate neuronal activity to attention or sleep or anger the cells in most of the brain show little predictable change, some of them are more active and some less active and we can only examine a few at a time. On the other hand, we know some of the lines of communication, and we have learnt so much already about the neuronal activity in the visual and tactile receiving areas of the cortex and in the cerebellum that it may not prove difficult to go one stage further. After that we can only guess.

At all events, our labour, wherever it leads, has been greatly assisted by Herbert Jasper. He is one of the pioneers who has helped us to clear the path through the forest as well as a chief organizer in the whole operation. If it ends by leading us out into open country we shall certainly need new maps of the natural world, new ways of thinking about it and about what we are doing inside it. It will be a triumph for neurophysiology, but I am not altogether convinced that we shall be the happier as well as the wiser for what we shall learn. So I will end with the well-known quotation from Louis Stevenson: "To travel hopefully is a better thing than to arrive and the true success is to labour".

Herbert Jasper has played an indispensable part in our labour and we have met tonight to show him how grateful we are.

ADRIAN

Herbert Jasper

Montréal est une ville unique en son genre. Canadienne-française et cosmopolite à la fois, elle ne ressemble à aucune autre.

Dans le vaste domaine des sciences neurologiques, nous avons réussi à créer un climat d'égalité et de fraternité et y former un cercle de chercheurs unis par un esprit commun de discipline scientifique. Mais c'est Herbert Jasper surtout qui a prêché l'évangile en terre étrangère, si je puis m'exprimer ainsi, et qui, renversant les barrières entre Français et Anglais a donné à ce cercle ses dimensions internationales.

It was Herbert Jasper who led in the move to establish a common cause with all the other nations of the world—the United States, France, Britain, the Soviet Union, Japan, Germany. The International Brain Research Organization has opened the way for the future. Man must learn to understand his own spirit and the working of his brain if he would save this world and so live at peace with himself and his neighbours.

And now I shall be personal and tell you how Herbert Jasper came aboard the Montreal Neurological Enterprise. I must explain that my own career became what it was because of the woman who became my wife and because of the professionals I met and joined at the crossroads of life. Destiny, it has seemed to me, stood at those crossroads. Most important professionally, I suppose, were William Cone and Herbert Jasper. Cone, a brilliant young neuropathologist, joined me at the Presbyterian Hospital in New York. Indeed, he was waiting, quite by chance it seemed, in my first little laboratory when I returned in 1924 from six months sabbatical leave in Spain. We went along together for a time, following the road a neurosurgeon must take, and trying to solve many problems of neurology with microscope and spanish metallic methods.

It was 13 years later, in 1937, when my path crossed that of Herbert Jasper. The scene had changed. We had moved to Montreal with our laboratory of neuropathology. We had many colleagues in our bilingual city. McGill University had built a neurological institute and opened it in 1934. What was needed in our growing neurological group was an electrophysiologist but I did not know it. I did not know that there was such a thing. At that time, we had helped to introduce radical operations for focal epilepsy. We made our localization by neurological examination, the story of the fits, careful X–ray study, air encephalography. These things seemed enough. Epilepsy had opened the doors of the operating room at the M.N.I. to a study of physiology of the brain in conscious man. I could, at last, do some of the things for man that I had dreamed of doing when a student in Charles Sherrington's Mammalian Laboratory of Physiology. We could question what Sherrington would have called the "preparation", and listen to his answer. What a future it seemed to open!–for anatomy and physiology and psychology.

In the Autumn of 1937, I gave a talk at Brown University in Providence, Rhode Island, on the invitation of Leonard Carmichael. He was then a neurobiologist who became President of Brown. He and Dr. Ruggles, the Director of the Bradley Home for retarded children, were promoting neurological work in Providence. I spent the night at the Bradley Home in East Providence after the talk and in the morning Ruggles said, "You must come over to the laboratory. There is a young man there who did his doctorate thesis on the electrical activity of the nervous system of crustacea, working with Lapicque in Paris. Now he is here on a Rockefeller-financed project to study human beings. He wants to talk to you". We made our way to an adjacent building. In the basement, there was a maze of chicken-wire. It served, I was told, as an electrical shield.

Inside the maze was a young man, moving about like a bird in an aviary. This was a rare bird, a *rara avis*, Herbert Jasper, a young man driven by one creative idea after another. He could, he said, localize the focus of an epileptic seizure by the disturbance of brain rhythms outside the skull. I doubted that but hoped it might be true. He wanted me to suggest to him the best young neurosurgeon so that they could invite him to come to Providence to help them build up a neurological centre. He had two patients suffering from epilepsy in whom he had localized the source of the trouble. He wanted to send them to Montreal right away for operation. In general, I wanted proof. He wanted the chance to prove and the chance to work in a clinical stream of medical science.

But memory is treacherous and so, when Professor Cordeau asked me to speak here, I turned to my Jasper file. The first letter that I could find was written about two months later on January 31, 1938. It evidently followed a visit he made to Montreal. It refers to "Eva Cyr" and "the Carozza boy," the patients he had sent to me in Montreal and on whom he had watched me operate. He expressed his thanks and added the following: "In fact, I was so well pleased with the entire setup that I could not help but wish that my own research team and laboratories were a part of your organization". Later in the letter, he says "I am very much interested in your suggestion that we collaborate in electro-encephalographic and neurosurgical exploration. After further consideration of the practical aspects of such a collaboration in the immediate future, it appears to me that it might be more satisfactory to do all that we can in order to complete your own technical setup as quickly as possible — I feel as though this is an extremely important project both from the clinical and the surgical points of view and we cannot afford to allow financial or other difficulties to interfere in carrying it through". Here we were certainly of one mind, Jasper and I—never to let financial caution hold one back!

My reply was written on the 7th of February. I had evidently already submitted a plan to Alan Gregg, hoping the Rockefeller Foundation would finance the collaboration we meant to carry out. But Herbert had not waited for my reply, for he wrote on February 5th: "I feel that this is such an excellent opportunity that you have suggested that I would like very much to spend the next 3 months in Montreal. But I do not see how that can be arranged in the immediate future". He then suggested the possiblility of travelling back and forth and added: "In regard to equipment, I have a very good portable setup which could be very easily transported to Montreal in my car".

This *"rara avis"* moved fast. But he was not only interested in gadgetry and electricity. The whole field of neurophysiology was to be his.

On March 10th 1938, he wrote about a visit he had made to Dusser de Barenne and others in New Haven. He observed that "the continuous pH determinations both of the circulating blood and of the interstitial fluid of the brain, being done by de Barenne and his colleagues, are extremely important. They are", he concluded, "particularly important it seems to me in relation to your blood flow findings and your theoretical interpretation of the mechanisms of epileptic discharge. I am convinced that the solution of the problem of epilepsy will not be found entirely along the lines of the rate regulators as indicated from the studies of Gibbs and Lennox. But, with their very important contributions, together with the work you are doing, which I hope to have part in, it seems that we are gradually closing in on the problem of epilepsy". This letter was written after he and I had instituted our almost unthinkable commuters' research project. It was as though far-away Rhode Island were a suburb of Montreal. He would arrive each week, ordinarily late Monday night, with his electrograph on the front seat of his car, and went to bed in a resident's room in the Institute. I would operate on a focal epileptic patient Tuesday morning and possibly another on Wednesday and Thursday. Friday, he was somehow back in Providence where he carried out a full week's work, discharging his responsibilities at the Bradley Home over the weekend.

From the very foundation of the Institute in 1934, we had organized a ski weekend for staff and fellows in the Laurentians. He attended this and we discovered the fact that Herbert Jasper had a weakness, a passion for the out-of-doors, for skiing, and as we were to discover later, for sailing and pursuit of the elusive ground hog. In a postscript to the March 10th letter, he added: "I am enclosing a few photographs of our ski weekend. This was a memorable occasion for me". But then he added, "We are having delightful spring weather down here in God's country, which provides an interesting contrast to Montreal. It was particularly impressive the other day to drive down the banks of the Hudson on a bright balmy spring day only a few hours after crawling through the snow in Montreal".

There is a later letter in the file that I wrote to him on May 10th: "I have managed to get hold of $16,000 out of the total of $66,000 requested for the 4 year plan of attack on epilepsy and psychosis. The Rockefeller decision will be made the 20th of May". Then, "I suppose you have heard of the almost fatal accident that has come to Ted Erickson. He is hoping you may come up for his wedding to Molly Harrower, as we all do". I added, "In case they [The Rockefeller Foundation] are favourable, I look forward with the greatest pleasure to our cooperation". I stopped in New York to see Alan Gregg a few days later on my way to the meeting of the American Neurological Association. Gregg said "Yes" and suggested that the Rockefeller Foundation would be glad to give another $25,000 toward the building of an electroencephalographic addition, a "lean-to" to be added at the back of the Institute (so recently completed and, as we had thought, so complete) provided I could get the promise of a matching sum from Montreal. So I telephoned to a new-found friend, a wonderful Canadian citizen—J. W. McConnell in Montreal. When he understood that the proposal would bring more Rockefeller money to Montreal, and that Herbert Jasper would come to boot, he exclaimed, "Why, of course! They must come. Go ahead". Well, we went ahead, and what fun it was! How much he added! And how delighted we all were when he and our own Margaret Goldie were married!

So we set up a laboratory of electroencephalography and joined it to our unit of neurophysiology. Then came the years of the Second World War and Herbert Jasper thought he would be of greater service in various ways if he were to add the M. D. to his other graduate degrees. He became a medical student at McGill. But he asked to be excused from none of his other duties. He still directed the EEG Department and he undertook added research that had its direct application to the problems of wartime aviation. It was a gruelling few years but he came through it strong and sane, receiving his degree in Medicine in 1943.

The years during which he and I prepared the manuscript of our book, *Epilepsy and the Functional Anatomy of the Human Brain*, were rewarding ones for me. Herbert Jasper understood. He helped me to think straight. We worked together week by week and even ran away to the mountains to write together. Each played his part on a wonderful team, the Montreal Neurological Institute. Many others joined us and each contributed what he or she could. They played different roles—Don McRae and Francis McNaughton and Ted Rasmussen and Brenda Milner and Peter Gloor, to mention only a few, and many that I see here tonight who now work elsewhere. I am grateful to them but I cannot judge the value of the achievement of each, nor of Jasper.

I hope when I pass on and people look at what I was, they will say at least: "This neurosurgeon became a neurophysiologist". It can certainly be said of Herbert Jasper now, that the electrophysiologist of Oregon and Iowa and Paris and Providence became a neurophysiologist in Montreal, a good one, a man of singular leadership. For 26 years, he made his own brilliant creative contributions to science at the Montreal Neurological Institute. On our professional team, playing the game of science and the healing art, Herbert was always loyal and always a leader. In 1964, he moved to the University of Montreal where his friend and former pupil, Jean Cordeau, could give him greater scope in neurophysiology. But the Director of the Institute would not let him go, not quite. And so Herbert works in both institutions. He has a special place in the hearts of all of us. We hold him there in deep affection and we pay our tribute to the achievement of this great Canadian with pride and admiration.

And now, in closing, let me say to our two good friends, Herbert and Margaret Goldie Jasper, 'Thank you, God bless you and grant you happiness and long life".

WILDER PENFIELD

La Photosensibilité Excessive du *Papio Papio*: Approches Neurophysiologiques et Pharmacologiques de ses Mécanismes

R. NAQUET ET Ch. MENINI

Département de Neurophysiologie appliquée de l'Institut de Neurophysiologie et de Psychophysiologie du Centre National de la Recherche Scientifique, 31, Chemin Joseph-Aiguier, 13-MARSEILLE, 9e (France)

Si mon ami et collaborateur Ch. Menini et moi-même présentons aujourd'hui ce travail, c'est parce qu'en 1954, j'ai eu l'honneur et la joie de travailler avec vous, Monsieur Jasper. Je me souviens toujours avec émotion des expériences réalisées en commun avec Ellen-Eva King à Long Beach et également de l'enseignement que vous m'avez prodigué en électroencéphalographie clinique et en épileptologie lors de mon séjour au Montreal Neurological Institute. J'ai gardé pour vous un profond respect assorti d'une amitié sincère et j'espère que l'exposé des travaux réalisés dans mon laboratoire depuis 1966 sur l'épilepsie est à l'échelle de tout ce que je vous dois. Vous noterez je pense au passage qu'à la naissance de cette série expérimentale on retrouve Ellen-Eva King devenue entre temps Mrs. Killam.

En 1966, Killam *et al.* ont mis en évidence l'existence d'une photosensibilité excessive chez une grande proportion de babouins *(Papio papio)* provenant d'une région du sud du Sénégal: La Casamance.

A la suite de cette découverte, tous les travaux réalisés sur les babouins ont confirmé l'analogie qui existe entre l'épilepsie photosensible du babouin et celle de l'Homme. Killam *et al.* (1967) ont même proposé de le considérer comme un véritable modèle expérimental.

Chez 60–80% des babouins provenant de Casamance, la stimulation lumineuse intermittente (SLI) à 25 c/sec déclenche des myoclonies des paupières qui peuvent s'étendre à la face, au tronc et aux membres. Ces phénomènes cessent généralement en même temps que la SLI, mais dans un plus petit nombre de cas, des manifestations critiques auto-entretenues peuvent se poursuivre après l'arrêt de la SLI et prendre l'aspect d'une crise tonico-clonique de type *grand-mal*. Un tel syndrome ne peut être attribué à des facteurs comme le milieu ou la nourriture puisqu'il a pu être observé directement dans le milieu naturel lors d'expéditions organisées au Sénégal (Serbanescu *et al.* 1968; Bert et Naquet 1969; Naquet *et al.* 1970). Cependant, la proportion d'animaux photosensibles est moindre (20%) dans le Sénégal oriental qu'en Casamance, et il semble même exister des différences selon la région, à l'intérieur de la Casamance, où les animaux sont capturés. Ceci semble indiquer que le syndrome photomyoclonique est une caractéristique de

References pp. 25–26

certains groupes de *Papio papio*, non de l'expèce ou du genre. Outre la photosensibilité, les divers groupes qui ont été étudiés se distinguent les uns des autres par des caractères particuliers: la distribution des groupes sanguins, par exemple, est significativement différente (Wiener et Moor-Jankovski, communication personnelle), il en est de même de la distribution des "red cell esterases" (Jolly et Brett, communication personnelle).

DISTRIBUTION TOPOGRAPHIQUE DES PAROXYSMES ELECTROGRAPHIQUES

Etude électroencéphalographique
Chez les animaux présentant les manifestations cliniques qui viennent d'être décrites, le tracé EEG comporte des décharges paroxystiques spontanées à type de pointes-ondes

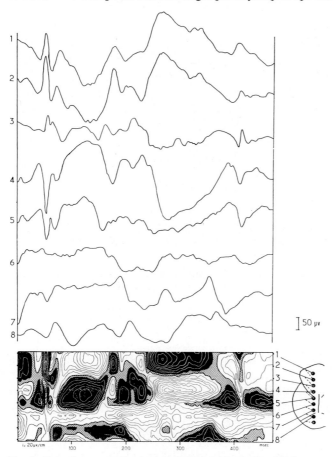

Fig. 1. Enregistrement électroencéphalographique d'une décharge paroxystique spontanée. 1–8: dérivations bipolaires jumelées, en chaîne rectiligne parasagittale. On remarque la pointe-onde dont la polarité s'inverse au niveau de la troisième dérivation.
    En bas: nappe spatio-temporelle correspondant à cet enregistrement. Les gradients négatifs sont indiqués avec un fond noir, les gradients positifs en blanc, la zone encadrant le zéro, en pointillé. L'intervalle entre deux courbes isogrades (i) est de 20 μV/cm (explications dans le texte).

(Fig. 1). La pointe, qui dure 10–15 msec et peut atteindre 150–200 μV d'amplitude, est surface-positive avec une localisation pré-rolandique précise; l'onde qui la suit, plus polymorphe, est surface-négative avec la même localisation. Les relations chronologiques et topographiques qui existent entre les divers éléments du paroxysme sont bien évidentes sur la partie inférieure de la Fig. 1: il s'agit d'une "nappe spatio-temporelle"[1] donnant une image tridimensionnelle de l'évolution des gradients recueillis le long d'un montage topographique (en ordonnée) et au cours du temps (en abscisse). On l'interprète, comme pour les dérivations EEG bipolaires classiques, en constatant que la zone d'inversion des gradients de grande amplitude correspond au maximum d'activité, c'est-à-dire pour la pointe-onde la dérivation 3. Ces pointes-ondes, synchrones des myoclonies lorsqu'elles existent, sont bloquées par l'ouverture des yeux et toute réaction d'alerte, elles sont favorisées par les baisses spontanées de la vigilance, en particulier lorsque l'animal a les paupières closes. Les décharges qui étaient au repos strictement localisées (Fig. 2), tendent, sous l'effet de la SLI à 25 c/sec, à irradier tout d'abord aux aires corticales antérieures et à la région sous-corticale immédiatement sous-jacente, puis à la capsule interne, au pont, à l'ensemble du tronc cérébral et finalement peuvent envahir secondairement toutes les structures profondes sauf le rhinencéphale (Fischer-

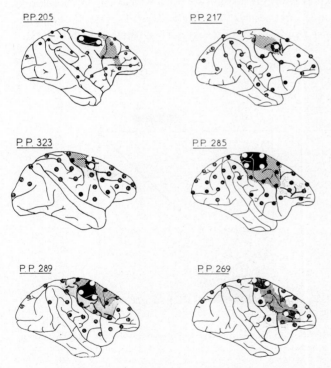

Fig. 2. Répartition topographique des points de départ des paroxysmes déclenchés par la SLI. P.P. 205 etc. = numéro du *Papio papio*. Il s'agit très généralement du territoire fronto-rolandique, rarement du cortex central (P.P.285) et rarement de la zone oculo-motrice (P.P.269).

---

[1] Réalisée par le Centre de Calcul du LENA, La Salpêtrière, Paris, France.

References pp. 25–26

Williams *et al.* 1968). Il existe une relative indépendance entre les régions antérieures et postérieures du cortex: les décharges paroxystiques occupent le territoire antérieur pendant que se poursuit, lors de la SLI, un entraînement dans le territoire postérieur.

Les décharges auto-entretenues qui se poursuivent après l'arrêt de la SLI débutent toujours dans les deux régions fronto-rolandiques, envahissent secondairement toutes les structures corticales et irradient à certaines structures profondes, notamment le thalamus, l'hypothalamus, la formation réticulaire et les noyaux gris de la base. Les décharges critiques enregistrées dans ces diverses structures sont toujours d'apparition secondaire et en relation avec la décharge fronto-rolandique qui prédomine pendant toute l'évolution de la crise. En général, le rhinencéphale n'est pas affecté par la crise et dans le cas où il est intéressé, c'est sous la forme d'une décharge critique indépendante.

Etude des activités unitaires corticales

Des enregistrements unitaires des neurones du cortex frontal ont été réalisés au moyen de micro-électrodes extra-cellulaires de tungstène (Menini *et al.* 1968b; Morrell *et al.* 1969) et comparés à des enregistrements simultanés de neurones occipitaux ou d'autres territoires. Il a pu être démontré que:

1. Les décharges paroxystiques sont plus facilement déclenchées par la stimulation lumineuse que par les autres modalités testées: lorsqu'elles sont absentes, le comportement cellulaire dans le territoire fronto-rolandique est normal, même pendant la SLI.

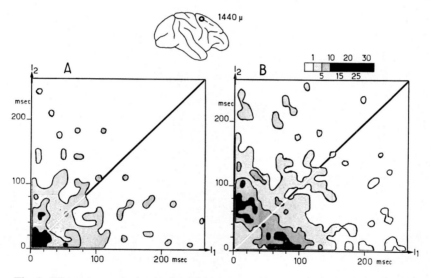

Fig. 3. Histogramme des intervalles-joints, pour une unité fronto-rolandique à 1440μ de profondeur. Blanc: absence d'intervalle. Grisé: la densité du grisé est en rapport avec la fréquence d'apparition des intervalles, le plus foncé étant la plus fréquente. *A*: activité spontanée. On note la prédominance des intervalles courts et leur groupement sur la bissectrice; ceci dénote une activité faite de bouffées irrégulières. *B*: au cours de la SLI à 25 c/sec. Deux maxima apparaissent, situés de part et d'autre de la bissectrice. A un intervalle I_1 de 80 msec environ, succède un intervalle I_2 de 10 msec, tandis qu'à ce dernier devenu à son tour I_1, succède un intervalle de 80 msec en moyenne. Il y a donc tendance au groupement des spikes par deux et à la répétition de ces "bursts" à une fréquence de 10–15 c/sec (donc sans rapport avec la fréquence de la SLI).

Cependant, l'un d'entre nous (Menini et Rostain 1970) a pu démontrer plus récemment que la SLI tend à produire une certaine synchronisation des décharges unitaires dans ce territoire, ou à la faciliter lorsqu'elle existe déjà (Fig. 3).

2. Il existe des relations étroites entre les activités unitaires et les décharges paroxystiques recueillies au moyen de macro-électrodes soit à la surface du cortex fronto-rolandique (Fig. 4) soit dans ses couches profondes. Cette relation ne se retrouve pas dans d'autres territoires (Fig. 5).

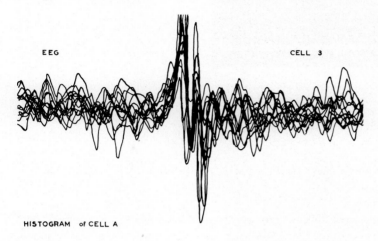

EEG   CELL 3

HISTOGRAM of CELL A

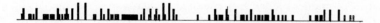

HISTOGRAM of CELL B   40 msec

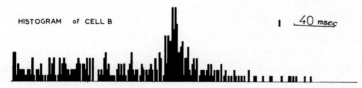

Fig. 4. Activation des unités fronto-rolandiques au cours des paroxysmes déclenchés par la SLI. *En haut:* paroxysmes électroencéphalographiques superposés. *En bas:* histogrammes de l'activité de deux unités fronto-rolandiques. La cellule B est activée de façon évidente, tandis que la cellule A semble au contraire inhibée pendant les paroxysmes.

3. Le mode d'activation des cellules frontales au cours des paroxysmes est très similaire à celui observé dans les lésions épileptiques focales rencontrées chez l'homme ou l'animal.

4. L'activation des cellules frontales ne peut être attribuée à une propagation dans un volume conducteur mais doit naître localement.

5. Spontanément ou même sous l'effet de la SLI, il n'a jamais été enregistré de décharge unitaire anormale dans le cortex occipital ou au niveau du champ oculomoteur (Menini et Rostain 1969).

References pp. 25–26

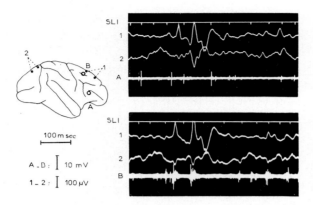

Fig. 5. Activation des unités fronto-rolandiques au cours des paroxysmes déclenchés par la SLI. 1 et 2: dérivations corticales de surface. *A:* unité oculomotrice ne présentant pas d'activation synchrone des paroxysmes. Il en serait de même pour des unités occipitales ou pariétales. *B:* unité fronto-rolandique présentant cette activation.

ETUDE DES ACTIVITES CORTICALES EVOQUEES PAR DIVERSES MODALITES SENSORIELLES

Potentiels évoqués visuels

(*a*) Au niveau périphérique, l'électrorétinogramme (ERG) peut être assimilé à un ERG de type I (c'est-à-dire d'une rétine à prédominance de cônes): une onde *a* négative, suivie d'une onde *b* positive très ample et très acérée, dans laquelle se différencie la déflexion photopique et scotopique. L'onde *b'* présente une négativité dépassant largement la ligne de base (Fernandez-Guardiola *et al.* 1968). Jusqu'à présent, aucune particularité de l'ERG isolé ou au "flicker" n'a pu être mise en rapport avec le degré de photosensibilité des animaux testés.

(*b*) Au niveau occipital, le potentiel évoqué visuel est très semblable à celui décrit classiquement chez l'homme, avec cependant des latences un peu plus courtes; la réponse évoquée est surtout caractérisée par une onde négative de grande amplitude à 40 msec de latence (Fig. 6, *A*).

La partie précoce de la réponse (20–80 msec après le stimulus) est maximum au voisinage de la scissure calcarine; la partie tardive de la réponse, amplifiée par la fermeture des yeux, intéresse l'ensemble du lobe occipital et est suivie d'une post-décharge rythmique non moyennable (Menini *et al.* 1968a, c, 1970). Il n'a pas été possible d'affirmer que cette post-décharge rythmique est en relation avec l'activité alpha occipitale du singe, cependant, elles occupent toutes deux le même territoire et réagissent de la même façon à l'ouverture et à la fermeture des yeux.

Le cycle d'excitabilité du cortex occipital a été étudié à l'aide de stimulations lumineuses couplées à divers intervalles. Il correspond aux données classiques: pour la partie précoce de la réponse, on constate une période réfractaire absolue de 20 msec, une période réfractaire relative jusqu'à 50 msec, puis une légère facilitation plus ou moins constante et le retour à une réactivité normale vers 500 msec après la stimulation. Aucune différence notable n'a été observée entre les animaux photosensibles et les

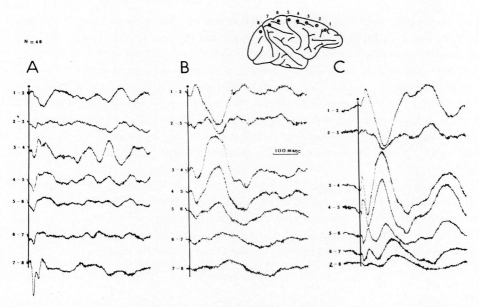

Fig. 6. Potentiels évoqués moyens recueillis en dérivations bipolaires le long d'un montage para-sagittal. *A:* stimulation lumineuse. Remarquer le potentiel évoqué occipital (7–8) et la post-décharge rythmique antérieure (3–4). *B:* stimulation auditive. *C:* stimulation somesthésique de la jambe contro-latérale: la réponse précoce est localisée aux électrodes 5 et 6; une réponse plus tardive et ample montre une inversion de polarité en 2–3, c'est-à-dire au même niveau que pour la réponse auditive et pour la post-décharge visuelle.

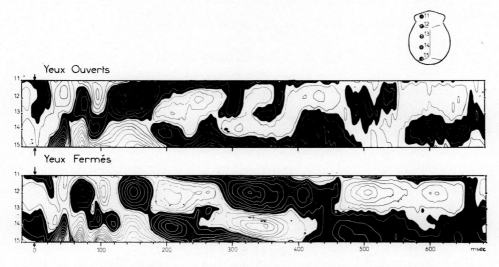

Fig. 7. Nappes spatio-temporelles de potentiels évoqués visuels (moyenne pour 50 éclairs) chez un animal très photosensible (Dérivations monopolaires). Les potentiels négatifs sont en noir, les positifs en blanc. Au niveau de l'électrode 15, on observe la traduction tri-dimensionnelle du potentiel évoqué occipital. Au niveau de l'électrode 12, une oscillation rythmique apparaît nettement vers 60 msec; elle est amplifiée et de plus longue durée lorsque l'animal a les yeux fermés.

References pp. 25–26

animaux non photosensibles. Cependant, l'étude des réponses évoquées unitaires permet
de penser que la SLI met en jeu des potentiels membranaires non propagés; elle ferait
par exemple, disparaître certains post-potentiels inhibiteurs (Menini et Rostain 1970).

(c) Au niveau du cortex fronto-rolandique: des réponses évoquées de faible amplitude et de brève latence ont été observées dans les régions rolandiques et oculo-motrices.
Les zones fronto-rolandiques se distinguent par la présence à leur niveau, d'une post-
décharge rythmique moyennable (contrairement à la post-décharge enregistrée au
niveau occipital). Cette post-décharge est très marquée chez les animaux les plus photosensibles et elle est amplifiée lorsque les animaux ont les yeux fermés (Fig. 6, A et
Fig. 7).

L'existence d'afférences visuelles vers le cortex fronto-rolandique a été retrouvée au
niveau unitaire mais seulement chez les animaux les plus photosensibles; les latences les
plus courtes ont été trouvées au niveau des couches corticales profondes. La latence la
plus faible est de 20 msec (Fig. 8), ce qui semble indiquer que ces afférences aient leur
origine directement dans le corps genouillé latéral ou le colliculus supérieur.

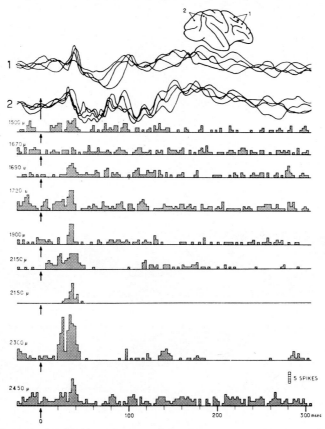

Fig. 8. Post-stimulus-histogrammes à la stimulation lumineuse réalisés pour diverses unités rencontrées au cours d'une exploration fronto-rolandique à l'aide d'une microélectrode. 1 et 2: potentiels
évoqués de surface. La localisation de la microélectrode est indiquée par une étoile sur la topographie.
Une réponse apparaît de façon évidente pour les unités situées vers 2000 μ de profondeur.

Enfin, les cycles d'excitabilité aux stimulations lumineuses ont également été étudiés dans le cortex fronto-rolandique; ils ont permis de mettre en évidence une caractéristique essentielle de ce territoire. Chez ces babouins, il existe une hyperexcitabilité trés importante, portant sur les éléments tardifs de la réponse évoquée visuelle à ce niveau, avec un maximum à 40 msec après la stimulation. Cette hyperexcitabilité ne se manifeste que lorsque les animaux ont les yeux fermés; elle est de l'ordre de 200–300% chez les animaux non photosensibles et atteint 600–700% chez les plus photosensibles. Elle se traduit par l'apparition d'une activité tardive oscillante localisée au territoire fronto-rolandique, particulièrement nette lorsque l'intervalle de stimulation est de 40 msec (Fig. 9), c'est-à-dire lorsqu'il correspond à la fréquence de stimulation la plus épileptogène chez cet animal (25 c/sec).

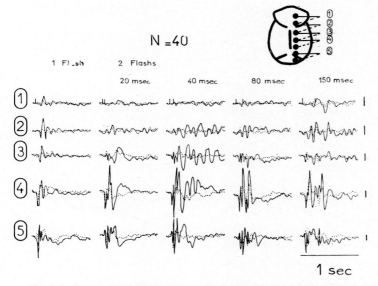

Fig. 9. Potentiels évoqués visuels moyens pour des stimulations lumineuses isolées (à gauche) et couplées à divers intervalles: 20, 40, 80 et 150 msec. Une post-décharge rythmique est observée au niveau des dérivations 2 et 3, pour un intervalle de stimulation de 40 msec; elle traduit une hyperexcitabilité très importante de ce territoire.

Potentiels évoqués par d'autres modalités sensorielles
Stimulations auditives. En dehors de la réponse spécifique que nous n'avons pas recherchée, on enregistre une réponse stable et moyennable dans la région pré-rolandique (Fig. 6, *B*). On distingue une onde négative peu visible à 15 msec, une onde positive à 35 msec, enfin, une onde négative très importante à 100 msec. Le foyer d'activité évoquée à ce niveau persiste jusque vers 500 msec (Menini *et al.* 1968c).

Stimulations somesthésiques. La réponse la plus précoce (14 msec) se localise dans la région post-rolandique controlatérale, où elle est suivie d'une onde négative à 38 msec. Au niveau pré-rolandique, une activité évoquée se manifeste sur les deux hémisphères dès 38 msec et persiste parfois plus de 500 msec. Toutes les composantes de la réponse, hormis l'onde à 14 msec, se retrouvent pour une stimulation ipsilatérale (Fig. 6, *C*).

References pp. 25–26

Il est intéressant de constater que des afférences de diverses modalités sensorielles (visuelles, auditives, somesthésiques) convergent au niveau fronto-rolandique. Cette convergence a été retrouvée au niveau unitaire (Fig. 10) et il est à noter que les unités qui montraient cette convergence étaient par ailleurs activées lors des paroxysmes.

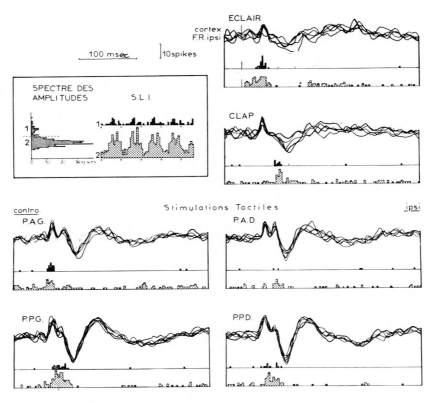

Fig. 10. Etude d'un groupe d'unités fronto-rolandiques à 2150 µ de profondeur enregistrées simultanément à l'aide d'une micro-électrode de tungstène. Dans le cadre: spectre des amplitudes permettant de dissocier les deux unités qui seront analysées séparément. Le post-stimulus-histogramme au cours de la SLI montre un entraînement des deux unités. Pour chacune des autres parties de l'image ont été représentés, en haut: le potentiel évoqué recueilli sur le cortex fronto-rolandique homolatéral à la microélectrode; en dessous: le post-stimulus-histogramme pour chaque unité.

DISCUSSION

Bien que la convergence hétéro-sensorielle ait lieu précisément dans le territoire où les paroxysmes ont leur origine, il n'est pas encore possible d'affirmer que la photosensibilité particulière de certains singes est dûe à l'existence ou à l'exagération d'afférences visuelles vers le cortex fronto-rolandique (Naquet 1969). Cependant, chez les *Papio papio* les plus photosensibles et en l'absence de toute drogue, on peut penser que la stimulation lumineuse engendre, par un mécanisme de "feed-back", un excès d'afférences multisensorielles vers le cortex fronto-rolandique; ces afférences agiraient au niveau de structures capables d'autorythmicité et d'hypersynchronie. Plusieurs arguments militent en faveur de cette hypothèse: d'une part les paroxysmes et les crises spontanées ou provoquées par la SLI débutent toujours au niveau fronto-rolandique et jamais au niveau occipital; d'autre part, chez la plupart des animaux photosensibles, l'injection de curare diminue la fréquence d'apparition des paroxysmes et empêche celle des décharges critiques auto-entretenues (Fischer-Williams *et al.* 1968).

Si les afférences multisensorielles jouent vraisemblablement un rôle important dans le déclenchement des décharges critiques, il faut cependant admettre qu'elles n'ont pas toutes la même valeur. Ainsi, la combinaison des stimulations lumineuses et auditives ne facilite pas l'apparition des paroxysmes; les afférences somesthésiques seraient donc plus efficaces. Et parmi les afférences somesthésiques, celles qui ont une origine péri-oculaire seraient les plus actives: si par injection locale de xylocaïne, on bloque les afférences provenant des paupières, les manifestations paroxystiques cliniques et même électrographiques sont considérablement diminuées (Ames et Naquet, communication personnelle) (Fig. 11). Des études sont en cours afin de tester si cette action est périphérique et ou centrale.

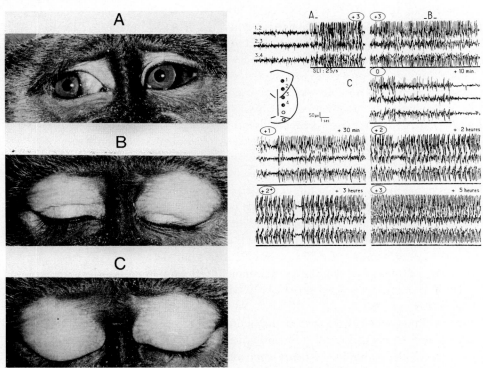

Fig. 11. Importance des afférences somesthésiques peri-oculaires dans le déclenchement des paroxysmes électrographiques au cours de la SLI. *A:* contrôle. L'animal photosensible n'a subi aucune manipulation; les paroxysmes sont d'apparition facile et s'accompagnent de myoclonies (+3, selon la classification de Killam *et al.* 1967). *B:* injection de sérum physiologique dans les paupières: la photosensibilité n'est pas modifiée. *C:* anesthésie locale par injection de xylocaïne dans les paupières; les décharges paroxystiques électrographiques diminuent en amplitude et en fréquence. Les myoclonies disparaissent totalement pendant 10 min (0); elles récupèrent progressivement entre 3 et 5 h.

References pp. 25–26

En dehors des afférences multisensorielles vers le cortex fronto-rolandique, la photo-sensibilité excessive des babouins doit être mise en rapport avec des caractéristiques fonctionnelles propres à cette zone corticale. Ainsi, des lésions destructrices unilatérales du cortex fronto-rolandique diminuent l'amplitude des pointes-ondes ipsilatérales et favorisent l'apparition de crises controlatérales, qu'il y ait ou non lésion du corps calleux (Catier *et al.* 1970; Catier, communication personelle). A l'opposé, si l'on produit une lésion irritative focalisée fronto-rolandique, un singe non photosensible devient photosensible, alors que des foyers dans d'autres territoires réduisent en général l'importance des paroxysmes fronto-rolandiques induits par la SLI (Dimov et Lanoir 1969).

Cette zone paraît donc se comporter comme un foyer épileptogène, mais étant donné l'absence de lésions histologiques précises à ce niveau (Riche *et al.* 1970), seuls des travaux pharmacologiques, histochimiques et ultramicroscopiques pourront peut-être donner une réponse. En particulier, l'incidence du syndrome photomyoclonique dans différentes populations de *Papio papio* suggère qu'une anomalie biochimique pourrait avoir un support génétique. Ces constatations nous ont amené à émettre deux hypothèses de travail: (1) l'anomalie biochimique intervient dans le métabolisme d'un neuro-transmetteur; (2) la décharge critique induite par une drogue doit simuler le plus exactement possible le syndrome naturel. Plusieurs drogues ont ainsi été testées:

L'ésérine et l'atropine qui modifient l'activité des systèmes cholinergiques sont inefficaces sur les réponses paroxystiques déclenchées par la SLI (Meldrum *et al.* 1970b).

La réserpine, qui provoque une déplétion de la sérotonine et des catécholamines cérébrales, n'agit pas non plus sur la photosensibilité (Balzano et Naquet 1970).

Les drogues qui modifient le métabolisme de l'acide gamma aminobutyrique (GABA), au contraire des précédentes, semblent efficaces: l'isoniazide et la thiosemi-carbazide diminuent le taux de GABA cérébral et facilitent l'apparition des paroxysmes; des crises peuvent même apparaître spontanément, c'est-à-dire en l'absence de SLI, mais elles ont tendance à débuter au niveau occipital et on peut penser que les crises induites par la SLI ne sont pas dues aux mêmes dérèglements biochimiques. Par contre, l'acide amino-oxyacétique, qui augmente le taux du GABA, bloque les réponses myocloniques. Ces résultats (Meldrum *et al.* 1970a) s'accordent avec plusieurs observations selon lesquelles l'anabolisme du GABA est plus important dans le cortex moteur qu'au niveau occipital, tandis que c'est l'inverse pour sa synthèse.

Certaines drogues hallucinogènes, notamment celles qui interviennent dans la mise en jeu de la sérotonine, bloquent la photosensibilité (Walter *et al.* 1971; Meldrum et Naquet 1971).

Ces résultats sont encore trop préliminaires pour permettre d'affirmer quel est le mécanisme pharmacologique ou biochimique responsable des propriétés particulières du cortex fronto-rolandique du *Papio papio* qui viennent d'être décrites; ils nous incitent cependant à poursuivre les études dans ce sens.

RESUME

De nombreuses études électrophysiologiques et neuropharmacologiques ont été réalisées sur des *Papio papio*, dans le but de trouver une explication à la photosensibilité excessive qu'ils présentent.

Du point de vue électrophysiologique

(*a*) Dans toutes les zones corticales explorées, sauf la zone fronto-rolandique, et dans toutes les structures sous- corticales étudiées à ce jour, aucune particularité fonctionnelle n'a pu être mise en rapport avec l'existence du syndrome photomyoclonique. Leur activité spontanée, électroencéphalographique ou unitaire, leurs potentiels évoqués sont normaux. Ces territoires, avec la restriction qui est faite, ont toujours été envahis secondairement par les paroxysmes électrographiques induits par la SLI.

(*b*) Le cortex fronto-rolandique se distingue par: (*1*) le fait qu'il présente le point de départ des paroxysmes électrographiques déclenchés par la SLI. L'activation de ses neurones, en relation étroite avec les paroxysmes, laisse supposer qu'ils naissent localement dans ce territoire; (2) la possession d'afférences multisensorielles et en particulier d'afférences visuelles dont la nature n'est pas encore déterminée. Ces afférences pourraient, par un mécanisme de "feed-back", mettre en jeu des afférences somesthésiques d'origine périoculaire et agiraient sur un système par ailleurs capable d'une certaine synchronisation; (3) une hyperexcitabilité aux stimulations lumineuses à la fréquence de 25 c/sec (c'est-à-dire la fréquence la plus épileptogène chez le *Papio papio*), cette hyperexcitabilité étant plus marquée chez les animaux les plus photosensibles.

Du point de vue pharmacologique

De nombreuses drogues intervenant dans le métabolisme des neurotransmetteurs ont été testées, sans résultats positifs à l'heure actuelle. Seules les drogues modifiant le métabolisme du GABA cérébral se sont révélées efficaces, bien que créant des décharges critiques différentes de celles du syndrome naturel.

Il est certain qu'une anomalie biochimique peut seule expliquer l'origine du syndrome photomyoclonique, et cette anomalie, qui n'a pas encore été trouvée, pourrait avoir un support génétique.

BIBLIOGRAPHIE

BALZANO, E. et NAQUET, R. Action de la Réserpine chez le *Papio papio* photosensible: modifications comportementales et électroencéphalographiques. *Physiol. Behav.*, **1970**, *5*: 561–569.

BERT, J. et NAQUET, R. Variations géographiques de la photosensibilité chez le babouin *Papio papio*. *Rev. neurol.*, **1969**, *121*: 364–365.

CATIER, J., CHOUX, M., CORDEAU, J.P., DIMOV, S., RICHE, D., EBERHARD, A. et NAQUET, R. Résultats préliminaires des effets électrographiques de la section du corps calleux chez le *Papio papio* photosensible. *Rev. neurol.*, **1970**, *122*: 521–522.

DIMOV, S. et LANOIR, J. Effets des lésions épileptogènes chroniques occipitales (cobalt-alumine) chez le *Papio papio*. *Rev. neurol.*, **1969**, *120*: 480–481.

FERNANDEZ-GUARDIOLA, A., VUILLON-CACCIUTTOLO, G. et NAQUET, R. Résultats préliminaires sur l'électrorétinogramme du singe *Papio papio*. *Acta neurol. lat.-amer.*, **1968**, *14*: 83–91.

FISCHER-WILLIAMS, M., PONCET, M. and NAQUET, R. Light-induced epilepsy in the baboon *Papio-papio*: cortical and depth recordings. *Electroenceph. clin. Neurophysiol.*, **1968**, *25*: 557–569.

KILLAM, K.F., KILLAM, E.K. et NAQUET, R. Mise en évidence chez certains singes d'un syndrome photomyoclonique. *C.R. Acad. Sci. (Paris)*, **1966**, *262*: 1010–1012.

KILLAM, K.F., KILLAM, E.K. and NAQUET, R. An animal model of light sensitive epilepsy. *Electroenceph. clin. Neurophysiol.*, **1967**, *22*: 497–513.

MELDRUM, B.S. and NAQUET, R. Effects of psilocybin, dimethyltryptamine, mescaline and various lysergic acid derivatives on the EEG and on photically induced epilepsy in the baboon (*Papio papio*). *Electroenceph. clin. Neurophysiol.*, **1971**, *31*: 563–572.

MELDRUM, B.S., BALZANO, E., GADEA, M. and NAQUET, R. Photic and drug-induced epilepsy in the baboon (*Papio papio*): the effects of isoniazid, thiosemicarbazide, pyridoxine and amino-oxyacetic acid. *Electroenceph. clin. Neurophysiol.*, **1970**a, *29*: 333–347.

MELDRUM, B.S., NAQUET, R and BALZANO, E. Effects of atropine and eserine on the electroencephalogram, on behaviour and on light-induced epilepsy in the adolescent baboon (*Papio papio*). *Electroenceph. clin. Neurophysiol.*, **1970**b, *28*: 449–458.

MENINI, Ch. et ROSTAIN, J.C. Enregistrements unitaires dans le cortex fronto-rolandique du *Papio papio* photosensible. *J. Physiol. (Paris)*, **1969**, *61*: 352–353.

MENINI, Ch. et ROSTAIN, J.C. Activités unitaires évoquées par la stimulation lumineuse dans différents territoires corticaux chez le *Papio papio*. *J. Physiol. (Paris)*, **1970**, *62*: 414–415.

MENINI, Ch., VUILLON-CACCIUTTOLO, G. et NAQUET, R. Etude morphologique, chronologique et topographique des potentiels évoqués visuels d'un cercopithecinae *Papio papio*. *Rev. neurol.*, **1968**a, *118*: 474–475.

MENINI, Ch., DIMOV, S., VUILLON-CACCIUTTOLO, G. et NAQUET, R. Réponses corticales évoquées par la stimulation lumineuse chez le *Papio papio*. *Electroenceph. clin. Neurophysiol.*, **1970**, *29*: 233–245.

MENINI, Ch., MORRELL, F. et NAQUET, R. Enregistrements corticaux au moyen de microélectrodes chez le *Papio papio* photosensible. *J. Physiol. (Paris)*, **1968**b, *60*: 498–499.

MENINI, Ch., VUILLON-CACCIUTTOLO, G. et LESÈVRE, N. Chronologie et topographie des réponses corticales évoquées par différents types de stimulation chez le *Papio papio*. *J. Physiol. (Paris)*, **1968**c, *60*: 277–278.

MORRELL, F., NAQUET, R. and MENINI, C. Microphysiology of cortical single neurons in Papio papio. *Electroenceph. clin. Neurophysiol.*, **1969**, *27*: 708–709.

NAQUET, R. Photogenic seizures in the baboon. In H.H. Jasper, A.A. Ward and A. Pope (Eds.), *Basic mechanisms of the epilepsies*. Little, Brown, Boston, **1969**: 565–573.

NAQUET, R., BERT, J. et GUILLON, R. Répartition de la photosensibilité dans trois populations de babouins (*Papio papio*). 3rd Int. Congr. of Primatology, Zurich, **1970**.

RICHE, D., GAMBARELLI-DUBOIS, D., DAM, M. and NAQUET, R. Microscopic lesions in brain in relation to the number of seizures in photosensitive baboons (*Papio papio*). Int. Symp. on Brain Hypoxia, Carshalton, **1970**.

SERBANESCU, T., BERT, J., GUILLON, R. et NAQUET, R. Etude de la photosensibilité du *Papio papio* du Sénégal oriental. *J. Physiol. (Paris)*, **1968**, *60*: 399–403.

WALTER, S., BALZANO, E., VUILLON-CACCIUTTOLO, G. et NAQUET, R. Effets comportementaux et électrographiques du diéthylamide de l'acide D-lysergique (LSD25) sur le *Papio papio* photosensible. *Electroenceph. clin. Neurophysiol.*, **1971**, *30*: 294–305.

Intracellular Microelectrode Studies at the Border Zone of Glial Scars Developing After Penetrating Wounds and Freezing Lesions of the Sensorimotor Area of the Cat

DANIEL A. POLLEN[1] AND EDWARD P. RICHARDSON JR.

Neurobiology Laboratory, Neurosurgical Service, and C.S. Kubik Laboratory for Neuropathology, Department of Pathology and Neurological Service, Massachusetts General Hospital, Boston, Mass. 02114 (U.S.A.)

It is a great privilege to be a speaker at this symposium honoring Dr. Jasper. His scientific achievements which have so enriched the neurosciences are known to all of us. No one in our field has had such command of both basic neurobiological research and clinical neurophysiology, and no one has so profoundly applied such knowledge toward a better understanding of the normal and abnormal brain. No amount of honor to him can repay our intellectual debts, nor sufficiently express the gratitude of those of us who have been privileged to be his students. At best we try to follow his example. And so today I wish to present some recent work bearing upon the pathophysiologic mechanisms of the focal epileptic seizure, an area so well-defined by Dr. Jasper (Jasper 1970) that if our work has any merit it is largely a credit to him and to Dr. Penfield who have charted the way.

During the summer of 1969 Dr. Trachtenberg and one of us (D.A.P.) were attempting to understand the physiologic function of the protoplasmic astrocytes of the cerebral cortex on the basis of the restraints imposed by our measurements of their membrane electrical constants. It was clear that the previously published estimates for the membrane constants of pyramidal cells (Creutzfeldt *et al.* 1964; Lux and Pollen 1966) made sense in terms of neuronal spatial and temporal summation properties (Jacobson and Pollen 1968) and their role in the generation of potentials recorded at the surface of the brain (Pollen 1969). It had recently been shown by marking techniques that the "silent cells" of the cortex were neuroglial cells which appeared to be protoplasmic astrocytes (Grossman and Hampton 1968; Grossman *et al.* 1969), and it was already known from work in other systems that neuroglial cells were electrically inexcitable and selectively permeable to K^+ (Kuffler and Nicholls 1966). Applying similar reasoning as to how cell structure, transmembrane ionic distributions and permeabilities determine internal and external current flows, we (Trachtenberg and Pollen 1970) came to the conclusion that the protoplasmic astrocytes were ideally suited to buffer the extracellular spaces adjacent to neurons and pre-synaptic terminals against the increases in external K^+ that accompany nervous activity. We had found

[1] Supported by Public Health Service grants NB-14353–04 and NB-08632–01.

References p. 41

supporting evidence for the possibility first raised by Orkand, Nicholls and Kuffler (1966) that at least one population of neuroglial cells served as " 'spatial buffers' in the distribution of K^+ in the cleft system".

No sooner had our calculations provided support for the spatial buffer concept than it occurred to us that a serious impairment of neuroglial function could lead to increases in K^+ around neurons and pre-synaptic terminals and an increase in neuronal excitability. In fact it had long been known and was now well quantitated that local increases in K^+ concentration could set off seizures in otherwise normal brain (Zuckermann and Glaser 1968).

Was a functional impairment present in the glial scars and meningo-cerebral cicatrices that are the histopathological concomitant of focal epilepsy (Penfield 1927; Foerster and Penfield 1930) and, if so, could an impairment in neuroglial function in long term fibrillary gliosis be the common factor in the development of the scar-related focal epilepsies? With this thought in mind and some histological and neuro-chemical supporting data from a number of workers, we (Pollen and Trachtenberg 1970) proposed a neuroglial impairment hypothesis that saw the neuron as the victim of fibrillary gliosis rather than as the primary agent in the focal epileptic disturbance.

That neuronal–neuroglial relationships might be an important area of study in post-traumatic epilepsy had already been suggested by Dr. Jasper (1970) who noted "since epileptic neurones act as though they lacked just such controls upon extreme and sustained shifts in their membrane potential equilibrium, and since this equilibrium is known to be controlled in large measure by ionic balances between the inside and outside of nerve cell membranes, one may raise the question of the possible role that might be played by the disruption of normal neuronal–glial relationships in the physiopathology of post-traumatic seizure tendencies".

A neuroglial impairment could come about in at least three ways: (1) by alteration of the normal neuronal–neuroglial anatomic relationship; (2) by either a primary metabolic defect or one secondary to vascular factors such that the neuroglial cell and its processes failed to maintain a very high internal K^+ concentration and restrict Na^+; (3) by an inability of glial processes to distribute K^+ over required distances if process "space constants" were significantly reduced as a consequence of their slowly progressive packing with gliofibrils. The first point has not yet been studied at the electron-microscopic level but some evidence supports the latter two possibilities, as astrocytes in established scars "show diminished quantities of glycogen and mitochondria" and "an extraordinary increase in the number of glial fibrils" (Maxwell and Kruger 1965).

We had hoped to soon put the hypothesis to a test but found no ideal animal model as most studies of convulsive activity have involved applying a toxic agent to previously normal neurons and neuroglial cells. The chronic alumina cream scars might have provided a satisfactory model, but we were more inclined the see whether any purely physical type of brain injury would lead to a scar and a discharging focus of "spikes" if not a frank convulsive activity.

Experiments were planned with three goals in mind. First, could chronic discharging foci be produced in the cat with either long penetrating wounds of the pre- or post-cruciate cortex or after freezing lesions to these same regions? Because we were doubtful as to whether penetrating wounds would produce a discharging focus, we sought for an additional method of injury, and Dr. Raymond Adams suggested the freezing lesion.

Our second goal was to provide a test of the neuroglial impairment hypothesis should any discharging foci be obtained. The expected consequence of neuroglial impairment would be a pile-up of K+ in the extracellular spaces, and we required an indicator for extracellular K+. For this purpose we decided to follow the changes of the undershoot of the action potential with repetitive firing after the method first employed by Frankenhaeuser and Hodgkin (1956) in the squid axon and more recently by Baylor and Nicholls (1969) in leech sensory neurons. That the undershoot of neocortical neurons is K+ sensitive has not yet been directly shown but is highly likely on the basis of other undershoots thus far studied.

The third goal was to see whether our test situation would be sufficiently worthwhile and practical to justify later attempts in cases of human focal epilepsy at the time of operation because epilepsy in man is not only where our clinical concern lies but the disease appears in a highly developed form almost only in man, for which reason there is always the unsettling question of the applicability of the animal model.

METHODS

Ten mature cats were prepared under pentobarbital anesthesia, 30 mg/kg. A single burr hole was trephined over either the pre- or postcruciate gyrus, and the dura was opened and retracted. In five cats penetrating wounds parallel to the cruciate sulcus were made by inserting a blunt # 18 gauge needle 2 mm into the cortex and dragging it through the brain until a trough of 3–4 mm had been made. In five other cats a freezing lesion was made by applying a 3–4 mm pellet of dry ice to the cortex for 30 sec. (See also Laskowski et al. 1960). The dura was then retracted back over the wounds, covered with Gelfoam, and closure was completed. All cats were given one intramuscular injection of 600,000 U benzathine penicillin G suspension (Wyeth Lab.), and there were no post-operative infections or complications.

EEG recordings and microelectrode studies were carried out 167–274 days after injury. See Table I. The cats were again anesthetized with pentobarbital, 30 mg/kg. With the aid of a heating pad, rectal temperatures were maintained at 36–37 °C. Our usual methods for intracellular study of neurons and neuroglial cells were used (Lux and Pollen 1966; Trachtenberg and Pollen 1970). Additionally, the intracellular data were recorded at appropriate speeds for spike undershoot waveform preservation, 30 in./sec, on a Hewlett-Packard 3917-C (Sanborn) multichannel, magnetic tape recorder. Intracellular data were later replayed onto a Tektronix 565 oscilloscope at high amplification so that spike undershoots could be photographed and more easily measured.

The brains were first perfused with normal saline, then 10% formalin for fixation, and later embedded in paraffin and sectioned at 8 μ. The sections were cut in an unbroken series when this was necessary to visualize the lesion adequately. Adjacent

References p. 41

sections were stained with cresyl violet (CV), hematoxylin and eosin (H + E), and phosphotungstic acid hematoxylin (PTAH) for the demonstration, respectively, of cytoarchitecture, general state of the tissue, and extent of fibrillary gliosis.

TABLE I

SCHEDULE OF EXPERIMENTS

P indicates penetrating wound. F indicates freezing lesion. RAS indicates right anterior sigmoid. RPS indicates right posterior sigmoid. Dates are given in the order: month, day, year. EEG spiking is indicated on a scale of + to +++. Zero indicates absence of spiking; +, slight; ++, moderate; +++, would indicate intense spiking.

Cats	Lesion	Gyrus	Date Prepared	Date Studied	EEG spiking
1	P	RAS	11.25.69	5.11.70	0
2	F	RAS	11.26.69	5.13.70	++
3	P	RPS	11.25.69	6. 8.70	0
4	F	RPS	11.26.69	6. 9.70	+
5	P	RAS	11.25.69	6.10.70	0
6	F	RPS	11.26.69	6.10.70	0
7	P	RAS	11.25.69	8.20.70	0
8	F	RPS	11.26.69	6.11.70	+
9	P	RAS	11.25.69	8.26.70	0
10	F	RAS	11.26.69	8.19.70	+

RESULTS

General EEG and extracellular microelectrode findings

In the 6–8 month period before study, but after the lesion, none of the cats was ever observed by the animal keepers either to have had a seizure or to have been in a post-ictal condition.

At the time of the acute experiment, surface recordings were carried out before beginning microelectrode studies. In the penetrating wound series, no focal spikes were ever observed. The amplitude of the EEG was frequently reduced directly over the scar, and in a few cases small sharp positive potentials (Fig. 1, *A*) occurred near the scar which were not observed over the homologous portion of the opposite hemisphere. No long bursts of action potentials were found. Occasionally, a cell would fire 3 or 4 times in rapid succession at rates of 200–400/sec.

In the freezing lesion series, four of the five cats showed focal EEG spikes at the site of the lesion (Fig. 1, *B–C*). In one case (Fig. 1, *C*) a projected discharge to the other hemisphere was present. The EEG abnormality appeared against a relatively depressed background of activity. In the other three animals the spiking was less prominent (Fig. 1, *D*) and seemed to comprise an exaggeration of the spontaneous activity.

In the four animals with focal EEG spiking, bursts of 8–10 action potentials firing at frequencies of 300–400/sec were observed (Fig. 1, *E*). These bursting cells were, however, the minority ($<20\%$) of all cells encountered extracellularly. In fact the incidence of finding neuronal firing at all seemed much reduced compared to penetrations in the contralateral cortex.

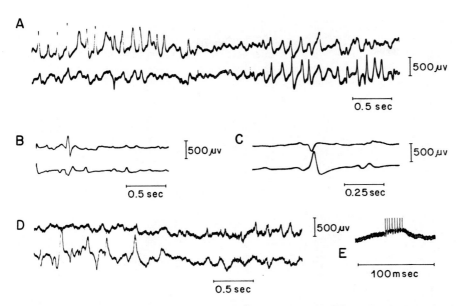

Fig. 1. An upward deflection represents negative polarity in *A–D*. In this and subsequent figures RAS, LAS, RPS and LPS mean right and left, anterior and posterior, sigmoid gyrus. *A*: surface recordings from LAS (upper trace) and from RAS (lower trace) close to penetrating wound scar. Cat 9. *B:* upper trace from RAS over freezing lesion scar and lower trace from LAS. Cat 2. *C*: faster speed of activity over RAS (lower trace) and projected discharge to presumably normal LAS (upper trace). Cat 2. *D*: activity from normal LAS (upper trace) and from region of freezing lesion scar RAS (lower trace). Cat 10. *E*: truncated action potentials showing bursts from border zone of a freezing lesion scar.

Neuropathological observations

The histopathologic appearance of each of the lesions was related to the way in which it had been produced. The penetrating lesions were slender and circumscribed as they passed through the cerebral cortex, then widened out in the white matter (Fig. 2, *A–D*). Surrounding the central cavity of the lesion, which represented the site of passage of the needle, there was a rather narrow border of fibrillary gliosis from which there was a rapid transition into brain tissue of normal structure. The freeze lesions, on the other hand, involved the cerebral cortex extensively (Fig. 3, *A–D*), and the adjacent zone of gliosis tended to be broader than with the penetrating lesions. In the zone of transition between the central portion of the freeze lesion, where there was nerve cell loss (Fig. 3, *A*) or cavitation (Fig. 3, *C*), and the intact tissue, there was a zone of less extensive damage to cortex in which apparently normal nerve cells could be seen surrounded by a meshwork of fibrillary gliosis (Fig. 4, *A*). Similar foci of gliosis containing intact neurons could be found in association with one particularly large puncture wound (cat 9, Fig. 4, *B*), but by comparison these were not as extensive or striking as occurred with the freeze lesions.

References p. 41

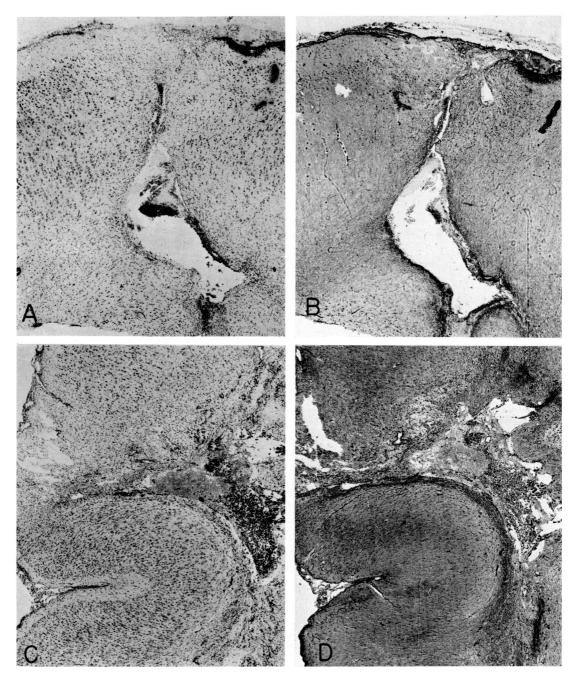

Fig. 2. Penetrating lesions. *A*: surrounding the central destruction in the cerebral cortex is a narrow zone of incomplete damage with rapid transition into normal cortex. The most extensive cavitation is in the white matter. Cat 1, CV, × 27. *B*: there is relatively little gliosis (dark-staining) surrounding the lesion. Cat 1, same area as *A*, PTAH, × 27. *C*: larger lesion than in cat 1, but damage to cortex is relatively circumscribed. Cat 9, CV, × 27. *D*: relatively narrow zone of gliosis at the border of the lesion. Cat 9, same area as *C*, PTAH, × 27.

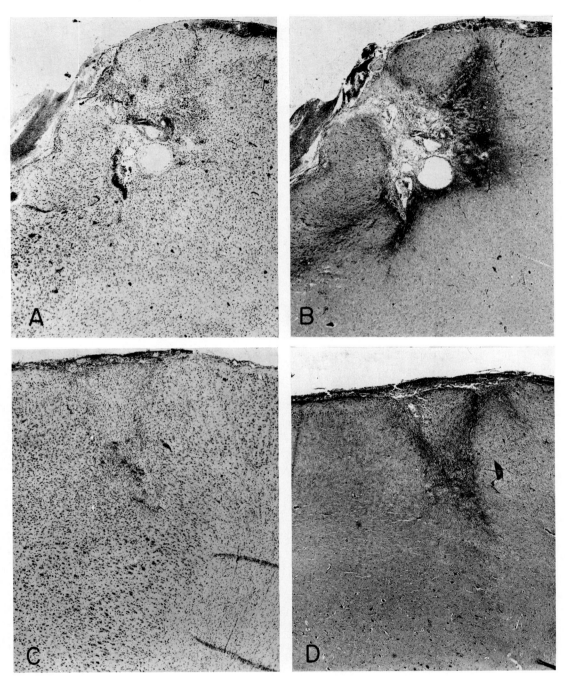

Fig. 3. Freeze lesion. *A*: extensive lesion involving a broad zone of cortex, with deep cavitation. Cat 2, CV, × 27. *B*: the lesion surrounded by wide gliotic regions which are situated in cortex. Cat 2, same area as *A*, PTAH, × 27. *C*: small lesion, but still extensively affecting cortex. Cat 10, CV, × 27. *D*: the gliosis which is in the cortex is conspicuous. Cat 10, same area as *C*, PTAH, × 27.

References p. 41

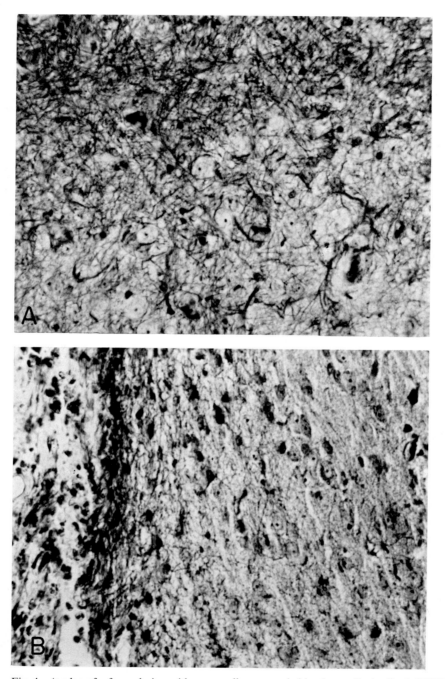

Fig. 4. *A*: edge of a freeze lesion with nerve cells surrounded by dense gliosis. Cat 2, PTAH, × 400.
B: edge of a penetrating lesion, with a narrow zone of dense gliosis near center of wound (left side
of illustration), outside of which are many intact nerve cells and a few astrocytes and glial fibrils.
Cat 9, PTAH, × 340.

Intracellular recording: general considerations

The greatest problem using micropipettes for intracellular recording resulted from frequent breakage of the fine tip of the electrode as it penetrated into the presumably scarred part of the brain. This was noted by a sudden drop in electrode resistance from 15–30 MΩ to less than 1 MΩ rendering the electrode useless for intracellular recordings. Tip breakage and the surprising paucity of nerve cells was previously noted by Atkinson and Ward (1964) in their alumina cream scar studies. To this we can add another irksome technical difficulty: the frequent plugging of the tip, often rendering accurate recording of the very fast spike undershoot impossible. The tip breakage problem was partially solved by moving away from the area causing breakage in 0.5 mm steps until an area which could be penetrated and still show focal abnormality was found. Nevertheless, we were able to carry out satisfactory intracellular studies in 4 cells in the penetrating wound series and 5 cells in the freeze lesion series exclusive of cat 2. Five "controls" were obtained from the presumably normal left hemisphere of the penetrating wound series.

All 14 cells were of the type well-described by Creutzfeldt *et al.* (1964) as showing a very fast rise time, a brief undershoot and a short after-depolarization variably followed by an even slower hyperpolarization (Fig. 5, *A–B*). After tetanic firing induced by

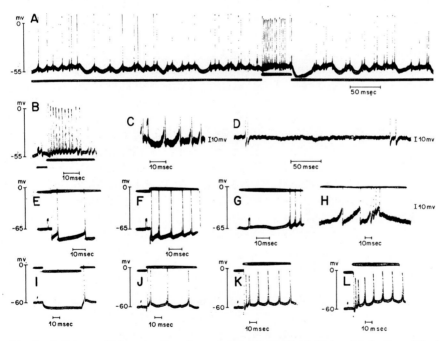

Fig. 5. *A, B*: intracellular recordings from a control LAS. Cat 9. Upward deflection of the lower trace indicates passage of current through the cell. *C*: higher magnification of spontaneous activity of same cell. *D*: "giant" extracellular spikes from LPS control side. *E, F*: action potentials after current injection to neuron in RPS of a cat with a penetrating wound scar. *G, H*: show spontaneous activity of same cell as *E, F*. Note progressive reduction of undershoot with repetitive firing with both injected current *F* and spontaneous activity *G, H*. *I–L*: hyperpolarizing and varying depolarizing current steps and responses from cell (see text) showing no spontaneous activity.

References p. 41

current passage through the microelectrode, very large amplitude hyperpolarizing potentials were observed (Fig. 5, *A*). It is not yet known, but would be of much interest to know, whether this very striking hyperpolarization resulting from the previous tetanic stimulation of *only the very same cell* resulted from firing a circuit involving an inhibitory interneuron such as is known to be brought into play when a bundle of pyramidal collaterals are excited (Phillips 1956; Stefanis and Jasper 1964) or whether it was produced by electrogenic activity or slow membrane permeability alterations. In any case these cells behave like the identified pyramidal cells previously studied by us with similar techniques (Lux and Pollen 1966) and considered to represent a population of "fast" large pyramidal cells by Takahashi (1965).

Two principal types of observations were made. In the first case the amplitude of the spike undershoot was measured as a function of the interval between two successive spikes evoked by varying rectangular current pulses through the microelectrode. As the threshold for spike firing varied by 1 to 2 mV depending upon the rate of rise of the depolarizing potentials, and because the very brief undershoot seems little affected in amplitude by these 1–2 mV variabilities, we found the most reliable way of measuring the undershoot was from the firing level. Plots of the amplitude of spike undershoot were then made as in Fig. 6. Undershoot changes would also be observed in "giant extracellular spike" recordings (Fig. 5, *D*) and undershoot changes seen by passing current were similar to those observed in cells firing spontaneously (Fig. 5, *A, C, G*) unless the depolarizing potential was quite large (Fig. 5, *H*).

If it is assumed that the undershoot represents a K^+ equilibrium potential and that most of the K^+ is leaked during the falling phase (and undershoot) of the action potential, then an approximate estimate of the increased extracellular K^+ can be made by using the estimates of Ames *et al.* (1965) for the normal intracellular and extracellular K^+ concentration in retina (as a prototype of a central nervous system tissue) and introducing a scaling factor to allow for the likelihood that the very brief undershoot either does not have "time" to reach K^+ equilibrium, or that extracellular K^+ is actually significantly increased before the maximal peak undershoot is reached. According to their data K_I is 142 mM, K_E is 3.6 mM. At 37 °C by the Nernst equation, an equilibrium potential of —98 mV would result. An estimate for the new extracellular K^+ (k) at a time (t) when an undershoot of $V_{K(t)}$ (mV) is obtained may then be made from the "scaled" expression

$$V_{K(t)} = \frac{^VK(max)}{98} \cdot 61.5 \log \frac{142}{k}$$

where $V_{K(max)}$ is the maximal value of the undershoot obtained for the "first" spike. These estimates for (k) are plotted at the right of the graph (Fig. 6) for a normal cell and one obtained near a penetrating wound scar. The peak added extracellular concentration at the shortest measurable interval after an action potential can thus be estimated as can the time for the added K^+ to drop to half its value. From the half-time a time constant (τ) (assuming an exponential fall) can be calculated, and in this way the K^+ fall-off for different cells can be compared. In the five normal cells, the half-time ranged from 1.8–2.8 msec and (τ) from 2.6–4.0 msec. In Fig. 6, *A* the extracellular K$^+$ added to the space adjacent to that where the undershoot is generated is close to 0.9 mM per impulse.

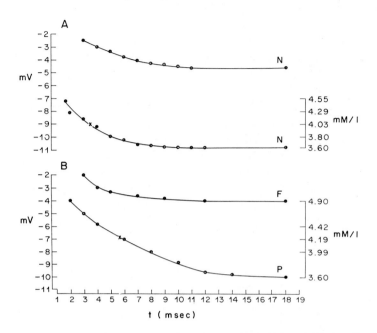

Fig. 6. Ordinate indicates amplitude of action potential undershoots. Horizontal axis indicates time (msec) between the first and second action potentials evoked by passage of current through the microelectrode. The two curves in *A* are from normal (N) cortices, LPS (upper trace) and LAS (lower trace). In *B* the upper curve is from an animal with a freezing lesion scar (F) and the lower curve from a penetrating wound scar (P). For the lower traces in *A* and *B* an estimate for the extracellular K$^+$ as a function of time after each action potential is plotted at right by the procedure described in the text. (X) on these curves indicates the mid-point between K$^+$ calculated for the earliest recording of undershoot after an action potential and the normal level taken as 3.6 mM/l. Half-time for K$^+$ fall-off can be estimated from graph from time at (X) minus time of highest external K$^+$ measured.

The (τ) values were essentially similar in all five of the cells from the freeze lesion scars (Fig. 6, *B*) and in all but one (Fig. 6, *B*) of the four penetrating wound cells. In this last case the (τ) value was 5.3 msec. We do not have a wide enough sample of normals to know if this difference is significant, but the second type of study suggests that it may be.

As a second test, the frequency of firing was observed after variable rectangular current pulses. Granit *et al.* (1966) have shown in the motoneuron how sensitive the frequency of firing is to small post-synaptic potential changes. If K$^+$ accumulated abnormally around a neuron, one might expect to find decreased adaptation or even a slight increase in firing frequency.

A decrease in adaptation cannot be documented as the pre-scar values are not known, but the opposite of adaptation has never been reported in normal pyramidal cells (Oshima 1969) and the finding would be strikingly abnormal. This was never seen in the normal controls, nor in the cells from the freeze lesion scar, but was seen in the cell near the penetrating wound showing the long (τ) value (Fig. 5, *F* and 6, *B*). Furthermore, the progressive decreases in the undershoot of successive spikes are particularly striking (Fig. 5, *F*).

In no cases were "epileptiform" bursts outlasting the period of intracellular stimulation observed, nor did we see any paroxysmal depolarizing shifts of the extremely large amplitude described by Matsumoto and Ajmone Marsan (1964) in drug induced foci.

One recording was made in a freeze lesion scar from within an excitable structure that showed no spontaneous activity, and had a very short membrane time constant (Fig. 5, *I*) and could be fired easily by depolarizing current (Fig. 5, *J–L*). The recording may have been from an axon rather than from a cell body, but the recording was stable for 15 min which would seem unlikely for a cortical axonal recording.

We also were able to record from electrically inexcitable cells with very short membrane time constants (<0.5 msec) in both types of scars. We cannot compare the resting potentials with those of neuroglial cells in normal cortex as in such a study we (Trachtenberg and Pollen 1970) arbitrarily selected only those cells with resting potentials of -50 mV or higher.

DISCUSSION

The first goal of producing a glial scar and a discharging focus by purely physical means has been a marginal success in the freezing lesion series. Though no seizures were observed, both EEG and microelectrode findings indicate that a hyperexcitable focus had been produced and the model could serve for study of the "trigger" if not the "propagation" problem in epileptiform discharge. Such differences as were observed in the extent of the lesion and subsequent neuronal loss and fibrillary gliosis are likely to be due to the variation in the technique used to produce the freezing lesions, and much improvement in our freezing technique would seem possible.

The difference in the EEG spiking produced in the freezing lesion series and the absence of it in the penetrating wound series is of interest. Though the lesions differ in a number of ways it would be tempting to interpret one difference as due to the presence of a relatively larger number of neuron cell bodies within a broader border zone of intense fibrillary gliosis in the freeze-lesion series as compared with the more abrupt transition zones in the penetrating wound series.

We do not believe that the intracellular findings in the scar area have provided much evidence either for or against the hypothesis of a neuroglial impairment in fibrillary gliosis leading to abnormal extracellular K^+ increases. Only one cell showed evidence of an apparently abnormal K^+ build-up in the surrounding extracellular space.

However, considering the microelectrode tip breakage problem when recording within much of the scar area, and the problem of being only able to find and record from a very small number of neurons close to the scar, the conclusion would seem to be that the intracellular technique may not be the most useful and appropriate for testing the hypothesis. Furthermore, the method we used would only test excitability in those regions where the spike undershoot is occurring and where most of the K^+ injected through the microelectrodes would be crossing the cell membrane. We were, therefore, not able to test for excitability changes as a consequence of a K^+ build-up along presynaptic terminals or upon relatively distant dendrites. In view of the large "dendritic" potentials comprising the primary surface negative part of the EEG spike, the "input" stage of the cell would seem to be the most likely place for the hypothesized abnormality to appear, though we have not yet been able to think of a satisfactory experiment to test this.

Probably the most interesting findings from the intracellular part of the study involve the estimates for the amount of K^+ liberated by a single neocortical action potential, and the rate of disappearance of the added K^+. Such data have not been previously available for a central mammalian neuron. Though the method of estimating the K^+ build-up (~ 0.9 mM/l per impulse) is only approximate and rests upon assumptions valid in other systems but not testable in the intact brain, it is interesting that it is of the same order of magnitude as around mammalian unmyelinated fibers (Keynes and Ritchie 1965) and leech sensory neurons (Baylor and Nicholls 1969). However, compared to these systems and also the squid axon (Frankenhaeuser and Hodgkin 1956), the time constant of the added K^+ fall-off of 2.6–4.0 msec is 10–25 times faster than the (τ) values (30–100 msec) reported in those systems. Such a rapid K^+ fall-off in the neocortex is striking experimental evidence and supports our theoretical treatment on the K^+ spatial buffering characteristics of neocortical neuroglial cells (Trachtenberg and Pollen 1970). Furthermore, the experimental demonstration of such a rapid K^+ removal system strengthens our belief that its severe impairment would be disastrous for normal neuronal function.

Our third goal to see whether our methods might be suitable for study of human epileptogenic foci at the time of operation remains in a gray area largely because of the microelectrode tip breakage problem and the small number of neurons encountered in and at the scar border as opposed to normal tissue. In any case, a more satisfactory way of testing the hypothesis than the intracellular method would seem to be in order.

In conclusion, we wish only to note that the importance in testing the neuroglial impairment hypothesis lies not simply in an academic point about a "mechanism", but rather in the point that a substantiation of the hypothesis might open the way towards an understanding and eventual control or prevention of whatever aspect of chronic fibrillary gliosis is deleterious. Nor does emphasis on testing the neuroglial impairment hypothesis imply belief in a "single-factor" model for post-traumatic epilepsy. Other likely factors, and in particular the importance of deafferentation hypersensitivity as brought out by Dr. Ward (1969), are considered elsewhere (Pollen and Trachtenberg 1970). Rather our interest is drawn to the fact that there has as yet been little attention paid to the possibility of pharmacologically modifying cortical glial scar formation (Clemente 1958). Perhaps also an understanding and correction of the genetic predispositions in focal epilepsy (Metrakos and Metrakos 1969) may someday be sought in terms of the biochemistry of neuroglial scar formation.

References p. 41

SUMMARY

1. Either penetrating wounds or freezing lesions were made in the sensorimotor cortex of ten cats. Gross potential studies, extracellular and intracellular microelectrode studies, and neuropathological studies of the glial scars and their border zones were carried out 5.5–9 months later.

2. No focal spiking was observed in the five animals with penetrating wounds, but occasionally neurons would fire 3 or 4 times in rapid succession at rates of 200–400/sec. Focal EEG spiking was present in four of the five freeze lesion animals, and in these animals bursting cells ($<20\%$ of all cells encountered) with 8–10 action potentials firing at frequencies of 300–400/sec were observed. The incidence of neuronal firing within the scarred area seemed much reduced compared to observations in normal contralateral cortex.

3. On histopathologic examination, the penetrating lesions were relatively circumscribed, with narrow borders of fibrillary gliosis. The zone of gliosis was wider in the freeze lesions and contained many intact nerve cells.

4. Attempts were also made to test the neuroglial impairment hypothesis by determining whether K^+ accumulated abnormally as a consequence of neuronal activity in the surrounding extracellular spaces within the glial scar border zone. Microelectrode tip breakage was a serious and often limiting technical problem in carrying out intracellular studies within the scarred areas. If it is assumed that the undershoot of the action potential of normal cortical neurons is selectively sensitive to the concentration of extracellular K^+, then each action potential (presumably of large pyramidal cells) adds of the order of 1 mM/l of K^+ to the adjoining extracellular space. Around neurons in normal brain the added K^+ rapidly disappears with a time constant of 2.6–4.0 msec. The experimental demonstration of such a rapid K^+ removal system strengthens our belief that its severe impairment would be disastrous for normal neuronal function.

5. In none of four successful intracellular studies in the freeze lesion scars and in only one of 5 cells studied in the penetrating wound scars was a probably abnormal slow removal of extracellular K^+ found.

6. Because of technical and sampling problems, the initial experimental test of the neuroglial impairment hypothesis as a factor in post-traumatic focal epilepsy should be considered inconclusive. Other theoretical and experimental aspects of the problem are considered.

ACKNOWLEDGMENTS

We wish to thank Miss Peggy Philson for her excellent technical assistance in all aspects of this work.

REFERENCES

AMES III, A., ISOM, J.B. and NESBETT, F.B. Effects of osmotic changes on water and electrolytes in nervous tissue. *J. Physiol. (Lond.)*, **1965**, *177*: 246–262.

ATKINSON, J.R. and WARD JR., A.A. Intracellular studies of cortical neurons in chronic epileptogenic foci in the monkey. *Exp. Neurol.*, **1964**, *10*: 285–295.

BAYLOR, D.A. and NICHOLLS, J.G. Changes in extracellular potassium concentration produced by neuronal activity in the central nervous system of the leech. *J. Physiol. (Lond.)*, **1969**, *203*: 555–569.

CLEMENTE, C.D. The regeneration of peripheral nerves inserted into the cerebral cortex and the healing of cerebral lesions. *J. comp. Neurol.*, **1958**, *109*: 123–151.

CREUTZFELDT, O.D., LUX, H.D. und NACIMIENTO, A.C. Intracelluläre Reizung corticaler Nervenzellen. *Pflügers Arch. ges. Physiol.* **1964**, *281*: 129–151.

FOERSTER, O. and PENFIELD, W. Structural basis of traumatic epilepsy and results of radical operation. *Brain*, **1930**, *53*: 99–119.

FRANKENHAEUSER, B. and HODGKIN, A.L. The after-effects of impulses in the giant nerve fibres of *Loligo*. *J. Physiol. (Lond)*, **1956**, *131*: 341–376.

GRANIT, R., KERNELL, D. and LAMARRE, Y. Algebraical summation in synaptic activation of motoneurons firing within the "primary range" to injected currents. *J. Physiol. (Lond.)*, **1966**, *187*: 379–399.

GROSSMAN, R.G. and HAMPTON, T.L. Depolarization of cortical glial cells during electrocortical activity. *Brain Res.*, **1968**, *11*: 316–324.

GROSSMAN, R.G., WHITESIDE, L. and HAMPTON, T.L. The time course of evoked depolarization of cortical glial cells. *Brain Res.*, **1969**, *14*: 401–415.

JACOBSON, S. and POLLEN, D.A. Electronic spread of dendritic potentials in feline Betz cells. *Science*, **1968**, *161*: 1351–1353.

JASPER, H.H. Physiopathological mechanisms of post-traumatic epilepsy. *Epilepsia (Amst.)*, **1970**, *11*: 73–80.

KEYNES, R.D. and RITCHIE, J.M. The movements of labelled ions in mammalian nonmyelinated nerve fibers. *J. Physiol. (Lond.)*, **1965**, *179*: 333–367.

KUFFLER, S.W. and NICHOLLS, J.G. The physiology of neuroglial cells. *Ergebn. Physiol.*, **1966**, *57*: 1–90.

LASKOWSKI, E.J., KLATZO, I. and BALDWIN, M. Experimental study of the effects of hypothermia on local brain injury. *Neurology (Minneap.)*, **1960**, *10*: 499–505.

LUX, H.D. and POLLEN, D.A. Electrical constants of neurons in the motor cortex of the cat. *J. Neurophysiol.*, **1966**, *29*: 207–220.

MATSUMOTO, H. and AJMONE MARSAN, C. Cortical cellular phenomena in experimental epilepsy: ictal manifestations. *Exp. Neurol.*, **1964**, *9*: 305–326.

MAXWELL, D.S. and KRUGER, L. The fine structure of astrocytes in the cerebral cortex and their response to focal injury produced by heavy ionizing particles. *J. Cell Biol.*, **1965**, *25*: 141–157.

METRAKOS, J.D. and METRAKOS, K. Discussion: Genetic studies in clinical epilepsy. In H.H. JASPER, A.A. WARD JR. and A. POPE (EDS.), *Basic mechanisms of the epilepsies*. Little, Brown, Boston, **1969**: 700–708.

ORKAND, R.K., NICHOLLS, J.G. and KUFFLER, S.W. Effect of nerve impulses on the membrane potential of glial cells in the central nervous system of amphibia. *J. Neurophysiol.*, **1966**, *29*: 788–806.

OSHIMA, T. Discussion: Studies of pyramidal tract cells. In H.H. JASPER, A.A.WARD JR. and A.POPE (EDS.), *Basic mechanisms of the epilepsies*. Little, Brown, Boston, **1969**: 253–261.

PENFIELD, W. Mechanism of cicatricial contraction in brain. *Brain*, **1927**, *50*: 499–517.

PHILLIPS, C.G. Intracellular records from Betz cells in the cat. *Quart. J. exp. Physiol.*, **1956**, *41*: 58–69.

POLLEN, D.A. Discussion: On the generation of neocortical bioelectric potentials. In H.H. JASPER, A.A. WARD JR. and A. POPE (EDS.), *Basic mechanisms of the epilepsies*. Little, Brown, Boston, **1969**: 411–420.

POLLEN, D.A. and TRACHTENBERG, M.C. Neuroglia: gliosis and focal epilepsy. *Science*, **1970**, *167*: 1252–1253.

STEFANIS, C. and JASPER, H.H. Intracellular microelectrode studies of antidromic responses in cortical pyramidal tract neurons. *J. Neurophysiol.*, **1964**, *27*: 828–854.

TAKAHASHI, K. Slow and fast groups of pyramidal tract cells and their respective membrane properties. *J. Neurophysiol.*, **1965**, *28*: 908–924.

TRACHTENBERG, M.C. and POLLEN, D.A. Neuroglia: biophysical properties and physiologic function. *Science*, **1970**, *167*: 1248–1252.

WARD JR., A.A. The epileptic neuron: chronic foci in animals and man. In H.H. JASPER, A.A. WARD JR. and A. POPE (EDS.), *Basic mechanisms of the epilepsies*. Little, Brown, Boston, **1969**: 263–288.

ZUCKERMANN, E.C. and GLASER, G.H. Hippocampal epileptic activity induced by localized ventricular perfusion with high-potassium cerebrospinal-fluid. *Exp. Neurol.*, **1968**, *20*: 87–110.

Fluids and Electrolytes in the Central Nervous System: Factors affecting their Distribution, with Special Reference to Excitability and Edema

DONALD B. TOWER

Laboratory of Neurochemistry, National Institute of Neurological Diseases and Stroke, Bethesda, Maryland 20014 (U.S.A.)

Ever since the concepts of metabolic compartmentation in tissues were revived by the late Heinrich Waelsch (1960), interest in and the importance of metabolic pools and compartments in the nervous system has continued to increase. Nowhere are the concepts more relevant than for fluids and electrolytes and their distribution in the central nervous system. In this presentation I shall discuss some of the factors which affect such distributions, especially as they relate to excitability (or seizures) and to edema (or swelling). Various aspects of these topics have long interested Herbert Jasper, and it is my great pleasure to be able to dedicate this paper to him.

Fluid spaces

There is little profit in continuing here the debate over the extracellular space of the central nervous system. The evidence is now rather overwhelming that there are in various areas of mammalian brain sizeable extracellular spaces. This evidence comes from the electron microscopic studies with freeze-substitution (Van Harreveld *et al.* 1965) and with ferritin (Brightman 1965), from neurophysiological studies on impedance (Van Harreveld and Schadé 1960; Fenstermacher *et al.* 1970), and from biochemical studies on the distribution of solute indicators *in vivo* (Rall *et al.* 1962; Reed and Woodbury 1963; Bourke *et al.* 1965; Woodward *et al.* 1967; Korobkin *et al.* 1968; Fenstermacher *et al.* 1970). One cannot and should not yet insist on absolute values, but even when one can, the absolute values will seldom be as important as relative values and comparative data. One would expect the size of the extracellular space to differ in various areas of the central nervous system. Data on this point are scanty but there are indications that the spaces in cerebral cortex, white matter and basal ganglia may each be of different sizes (Rall *et al.* 1962; Bourke *et al.* 1965; Ranck and BeMent 1965; Tower and Bourke 1966; Korobkin *et al.* 1968). Perhaps of greater importance is the fact that the size of the extracellular space of cerebral cortex differs from species to species (Bourke *et al.* 1965), as depicted schematically in Fig. 1. Despite some scepticism and the need for further verification, evidence in support of the correlation of cerebral cortical extracellular space with species brain size is accumulating. The value for inulin space of rat cerebral cortex of 14.5% predicted by extrapolation (Bourke *et al.* 1965) has been verified by direct measurements (Woodward *et al.* 1967), and the value of 24% for sucrose space of cat cerebral cortex reported by Korobkin *et al.* (1968) is very close to the value of 27% originally reported by Bourke *et al.* (1965). One of the parameters included in the correlations depicted by Fig. 1 is the content of chloride in cerebral cortex. Recently we have been able to measure this in cerebral cortex of the fin whale *(Balaenoptera physalus)*. The measure value of 64.8 μequiv/g wet weight (Young, O. M. and Tower, D. B., unpublished data) is very close to the value of 67.3 originally predicted by extrapolation (Bourke *et al.* 1965). These examples provide further confidence that the original correlations schematized in Fig. 1 are indeed valid. Hence the factors of variation among species and among brain regions within a species are important in any consideration of the distribution of fluid between extracellular and intracellular compartments of the central nervous system.

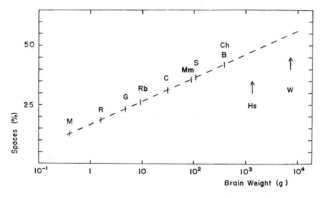

Fig. 1. Schematic summary of the correlation between cortical fluid spaces (*ordinate*) and species brain size (*abscissa*, log scale). The plot is approximated from the individual curves for the fluid spaces in cerebral cortex accessible *in vivo* to inulin, sucrose, chloride and thiocyanate (Bourke *et al.* 1965). Species for which one or more sets of data were obtained are indicated by small vertical lines intersecting the curve. Key to species: *M*, mouse; *R*, rat; *G*, guinea pig; *Rb*, rabbit; *C*, cat; *Mm*, monkey, *S*, sheep; *Ch*, chimpanzee; *B*, beef. The predicted positions for man (*Hs*) and whale (*W*) on the curve are indicated. (Reproduced from Fig. 1 in Tower 1967.)

Edema (or swelling) in vitro

One of the most troublesome and also one of the most important problems in the study of fluid distribution in brain is the propensity of the tissue to become edematous or to swell (*i.e.*, imbibe extra fluid) under a great variety of circumstances (Table I). Most of the well documented examples of cerebral edema *in vivo* are characterized by a predilection of the edema fluid for white matter, whereas in slices of cerebral tissues incubated *in vitro* it is the cerebral cortex which characteristically swells. The swelling *in vitro* of cerebral cortex from adult animals contrasts with the minimal swelling of corpus callosum from the same animal and with the total lack of swelling in incubated slices of neonatal cerebral cortex. However, in the presence of inhibitory concentrations of ouabain, both white matter and neonatal cortex will swell (Tower 1968), as one indication of inhibition of the cation pumps.

TABLE I

TYPES OF EDEMA IN CEREBRAL TISSUES

Species	Pathology	Cerebral cortex			Subcortical white		
		Dry wt. Control	% Exp'tal	Swelling (%)	Dry wt. Control	% Exp'tal	Swelling (%)
In vivo							
Man	Tumor	17.4	16.9	0	30.7	17.4	81
Rabbit	Alkyl tin	20.2	20.0	0	30.8	22.9	36
Cat	Freezing lesion	17.9	18.5	0	31.2	22.1	43
Cat	Circulatory arrest	16.0	13.5	18.5[1]	29.6	29.0	0
In vitro	(incubated slices)						
Adult cat	Incubated with 27 mM K^+	—	—	32.7[2]	—	—	6.7
	+ ouabain (10^{-5} M)	—	—	45.1	—	—	15.3
Neonatal kitten	Incubated with 27 mM K^+	—	—	(−1.2)	—	—	—
	+ ouabain (10^{-5} M)	—	—	19.6	—	—	—

[1] In perfused monkey cortex swelling is 22.2% after circulatory arrest but only 5.8% if the perfusate is Cl-free (Bourke *et al.* 1970b).

[2] In Cl-free (isethionate) media swelling is only 10–14%, mostly attributable to adherent medium (Bourke and Tower 1966a).

Data have been compiled from: Stewart-Wallace (1939); Aleu *et al.* (1963); Pappius and Gulati (1963); Bourke and Tower (1966a); Tower and Bourke (1966) and Tower (1968).

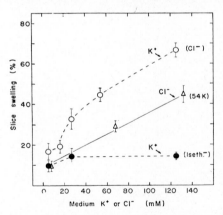

Fig. 2. Swelling of incubated slices of cat cerebral cortex (*ordinate;* percentage of initial fresh weight) plotted as a function of the concentration of K^+ and Cl^- in the incubation medium (*abscissa*). The curve with open circles provides data for slices incubated in a constant concentration of Cl^- (132 mM) but in different concentrations of K^+. The curve with open triangles depicts the converse, *i.e.*, slices incubated in a constant concentration of K^+ (54 mM) but in different concentrations of Cl^-. When the Cl^- of the medium is completely replaced by isethionate (Iseth⁻) the effects of different concentrations of K^+ on slice swelling are given by the curve plotted with solid circles. Standard deviations of mean values are denoted by vertical bars. The data have been adapted from Bourke and Tower (1966a) and Bourke (1969b).

We have studied in some detail the nature of this swelling of cerebral cortex *in vitro* and find that it is both potassium- and chloride-dependent (Fig. 2). Thus, the progressively greater imbibition of fluid that occurs as cerebral cortical slices are incubated in increasing concentrations of external K^+ can be almost completely prevented if the less permeable anion, isethionate, is substituted for the principal extracellular anion, chloride (Bourke and Tower 1966a; Bourke 1969b). If, as already indicated, the size of the extracellular space in cerebral cortex varies as a function of species brain weight (Fig. 1), why is the swelling of incubated cortical slices essentially identical, regardless of species, under the same experimental conditions *in vitro*? This apparent paradox can be partially explained by the fact that most of the edema fluid of the incubated slices is in a compartment or compartments not accessible to solutes such as inulin and hence is presumed to be cellular rather than extracellular in location (Varon and McIlwain 1961; Keesey *et al.* 1965; Bourke and Tower 1966a). On morphological grounds (Farquhar and Hartmann 1957; Gerschenfeld *et al.* 1959; Wanko and Tower 1964) and on the basis of biochemical characteristics (Koch *et al.* 1962; Nicholls and Kuffler 1964; Kuffler *et al.* 1966) the cellular compartment most likely to be involved is that of the astroglia. There is the intriguing observation (Tower 1967) that as the neuron density of cerebral cortex decreases as a function of increasing species brain size (Tower and Elliot 1952a; Tower 1954), the glia/neuron index increases (Friede 1954; Hawkins and Olszewski 1957). Since the calculated slopes of the two curves (Fig. 3) are of a similar order of magnitude, the density of glial cells per unit volume of cerebral cortex would remain essentially constant from mouse to whale. If this be so, and if this constancy applied to the astrocytes, then the constancy of swelling of incubated cortical slices *in vitro* would be understandable.

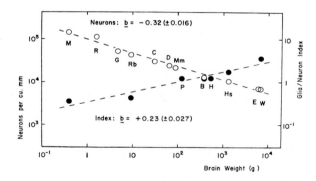

Fig. 3. Double logarithmic plots of the correlations of cortical neuron density (0) (*left ordinate*) and of glia/neuron index (●) (*right ordinate*) with species brain weights (*abscissa*) for various species. The curves were calculated by the method of least squares and the respective slopes, b (± S.D.), are indicated on the plot. Key to species as in Fig. 1, plus *D*, dog; *P*, pig; *H*, horse; and *E*, elephant. (Reproduced from Fig. 3 in Tower 1967.)

The distinction between cerebral edema commonly encountered *in vivo* and that characteristic of brain tissue slices *in vitro* is further emphasized by the differences in composition of the edema fluid itself (Table II). The edema fluid in cerebral white matter in association with tumors, alkyl tin intoxication and freezing lesions is characteristically high in Na^+ and Cl^- and usually contains appreciable amounts of albumin-rich proteins. Hence it resembles a serum exudate, as the pathological studies by Klatzo *et al.* (1958, 1965) clearly indicate. On the other hand the K^+ and/or Cl^- dependent edema of incubated cerebral cortical slices (Fig. 2) is characterized by edema fluid high in K^+ and Cl^- (Table II).

TABLE II

COMPOSITION OF EDEMA FLUIDS

Preparation	Swelling (%)	Na+ (mM)	Cl− (mM)	K+ (mM)	Albumen (g/l)
DOG: subcortical white matter freezing lesion	∼ 43	123.4	86.7	59.5	18.7
CAT: cerebral cortex incubated slices (54 mM K+)	∼ 33	39.0	135.1	107.5	—

Data have been compiled from Clasen *et al.* (1967) and Bourke (1969b).

In the course of studies on the mechanisms responsible for this latter type of edema, evidence was obtained (Table III; Fig. 4) indicative of mediated transport of Cl^- *into* the intracellular compartment in which this type of edema occurs. Since the apparent K_m for K^+ is one order of magnitude smaller than that for Cl^-, the concentration of K^+ rather than Cl^- appears to be the limiting factor in the inward transport of Cl^- into

TABLE III

MEDIATED TRANSPORT OF CHLORIDE IN CEREBRAL CORTEX *In Vitro*

Variable	V_{max} (mmoles/g/min)	K_m (mM)	Difference from Diffusion
External Cl−	7.7	245	$P < 0.02$
External K+	0.19	30	$P < 0.001$

Data were obtained on slices of cat cerebral cortex incubated with [36]Cl and various concentrations of Cl^- (37–138 mM) or K^+ (27–100 mM). Adapted from Bourke (1969a). See also Fig. 4.

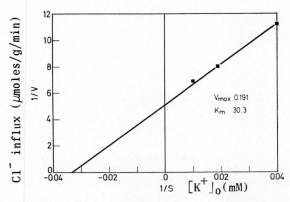

Fig. 4. Lineweaver-Burk plot of the reciprocal of the rate of influx of Cl^- (*ordinate*; 1/v) from the extracellular compartment into cat cerebral cortex as a function of the reciprocal of the external concentration of K^+ (*abscissa*; 1/s). (Reproduced from Bourke 1969a.)

48   D. B. TOWER

slices of cerebral cortex (Bourke 1969a, b). This observation, together with the composition of the edema fluid (high K$^+$, high Cl$^-$) encountered in such experiments (Table
II), strongly suggest that we are dealing with the mammalian equivalent of the high K$^+$
glial system described for the invertebrate and amphibian central nervous system
(CNS) (Kuffler and Potter 1964; Nicholls and Kuffler 1964; Kuffler *et al.* 1966). For
this system Orkand *et al.* (1966) have proposed that the inward transport of K$^+$ by
the glial cells provides a mechanism for the rapid clearance of K$^+$ from the immediate
extraneuronal environment following neuronal activity. In the mammalian system,
Cl$^-$ would presumably function as the anion associated with the movement of K$^+$
into the astrocytes (Bourke 1969b). It is pertinent that the concentration of Cl$^-$ in
cerebro-spinal fluid (CSF) and interstitial fluid of the CNS is apparently maintained
significantly above blood levels (Davson 1956; Friedman *et al.* 1963) by a system of
mediated transport of Cl$^-$ from blood to CSF with a location primarily in choroid
plexuses (Woodbury 1968; Bourke *et al.* 1970a).

Edema of cerebral cortex in vivo
Before the full implications of the findings *in vitro* on mammalian CNS can be considered, it is essential to know whether similar events can occur *in vivo*. When the surface
of primate cerebral cortex is perfused *in vivo* in a closed system (Lexan calvarium) with
artificial CSF containing various concentrations of K$^+$ or Cl$^-$ or both (Bourke *et al.*
1970 b), the occurence of K$^+$ and/or Cl$^-$ dependent edema of the cerebral cortex qualitatively similar to that already described for incubated slices of cerebral cortex *in
vitro* (Fig. 2) can be clearly demonstrated (Fig. 5). Thus, the findings *in vitro* cannot be
dismissed as artifacts associated with the incubated slice preparation. Presumably both

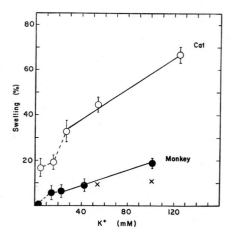

Fig. 5. Swelling of cerebral cortex (*ordinate;* percentage of initial fresh weight) of the cat *in vitro*
(upper curve) in comparison to that of the monkey *in vivo* (lower curve) both plotted as functions of the
external concentration of K$^+$ (*abscissa*). For these curves the external Cl$^-$ concentrations were 132 mM
and 129 mM, for cat and monkey respectively. The effects of reducing external Cl$^-$ (by replacement
with isethionate) to 10 mM and 12 mM, respectively, are illustrated by the $\times$ plotted directly beneath
the respective control values. Standard deviations of mean values are denoted by the vertical bars.
The data have been adapted from Bourke *et al.* (1970b).

the *in vivo* and *in vitro* K^+ and/or Cl^- dependent edema of cerebral cortex reflects similar mechanisms, very possibly the mediated transport system of the high K^+ glial cells already discussed. Because of the large reservoir of blood Cl^-, it is difficult *in vivo* to examine directly the mediated transport of Cl^- from perfusion fluid into cerebral cortex (Bourke *et al.* 1970b), so that this possibility can only be inferred by analogy with studies *in vitro* at this stage in our knowledge.

As already indicated (Table I), circulatory arrest is one of the few pathological situations in which the associated edema is preferentially found in cerebral cortex rather than in white matter. This type of edema can be minimized if the surface of the cortex (in the monkey) is perfused with Cl-free CSF during the circulatory arrest (Table IV) (Bourke *et al.* 1970b). The importance of this observation relates to the facts that there is significant leakage of K^+ from neural cells into CSF after circulatory arrest (Tower 1967; Bourke *et al.* 1970b), and that the extracellular (inulin or sucrose) spaces in cerebral cortex are markedly decreased, presumably as a consequence of cellular swelling, after circulatory arrest (Rall *et al.* 1962). On the other hand respiratory arrest or hypoxia does not produce analogous changes (Table IV), and Norris and Pappius (1970) have argued with some justice that the data on circulatory arrest represent postmortem changes since the length of circulatory arrest (15–30 min) seems unlikely to be compatible with survival.

TABLE IV

EFFECTS OF CIRCULATORY OR RESPIRATORY ARREST IN CEREBRAL GRAY MATTER

Conditions	Circulatory Arrest			Respiratory Arrest[1]
	Monkey[2]	Dog[3]		Cat[2]
	Swelling (%)	Inulin Space (%)	Sucrose Space (%)	Swelling (%)
Perfused control	0.7	12.7	18.1	—
Arrest (5–7 min)	—	—	—	3.8[4]
Arrest (30–60 min)	22.2	5.4	6.6	0[5]
Cl-free perfusate	5.8	—	—	—

[1] Respiration arrested until blood pressure failed (5–7 min) and then resumed with 100% O_2.
[2] Cerebral cortex.
[3] Caudate nucleus.
[4] $P < 0.02$.
[5] After survival for 1 hr.
Data have been taken from Rall *et al.* (1962), Bourke *et al.* (1970b) and Norris and Pappius (1970).

The problem posed here is of more than theoretical interest because it relates directly to situations encountered clinically in transient ischemic attacks and frank cerebral vascular occlusions characterizing strokes. If edema of the perivascular brain tissue accompanies such events, in a manner analogous to the edema of experimentally-induced circulatory arrest (Tables I and IV), there would be important implications for therapy during the immediate period following a cerebrovascular accident. Despite the rather compelling arguments to the contrary marshalled by Norris and Pappius (1970), the possibility of such edema cannot yet be dismissed for two reasons. One is the usually relatively localized nature of the occlusion clinically, a characteristic which makes assessment of the presence or absence of edema difficult. The other is the interesting observation made by Ames and colleagues of the "no-reflow" phenomenon or failure to re-perfuse localized brain areas after experimentally-induced ischemia of brain (Ames *et al.* 1968; Chiang *et al.* 1968). In these studies distinct areas failed to re-perfuse as a consequence partly of increased viscosity of blood in the involved vessels and partly of reduced calibre of small vessels from perivascular edema (Ames *et al.* 1968). The most important positive findings were swelling of the perivascular astroglia resulting in demonstrable compression of capillary lumina and the presence of cellular blebs (probably from swollen endothelial cells) in the capillary lumina (Chiang *et al.* 1968). These investigators believe that the neurons in such areas would survive a period of ischemia longer than 15 min if full re-perfusion could subsequently be achieved, and thus any irreversible necrotic changes would reflect the very much longer periods of ischemia secondary to the "no-reflow" phenomenon (Ames *et al.* 1968). Accordingly, they stressed that therapeutic measures should be directed toward a lowering of blood viscosity, elevation of the blood (or perfusion) pressure, and prevention of the swelling of perivascular glia (Chiang *et al.* 1968).

Ouabain and seizures
The original observations on the high K^+ glial cells were concerned with mechanisms

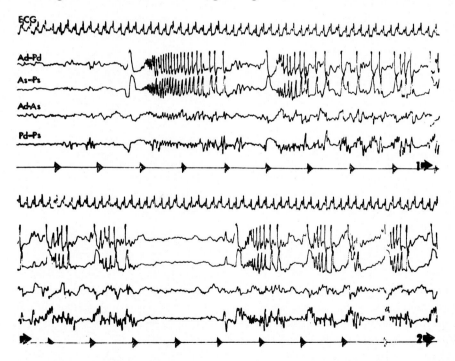

Fig. 6. EEG recorded with skull electrodes from a rat some 3 h after the intracranial injection of ouabain (0.4–0.8 µmole in 250 µl of saline). This is a selection from many different levels of hyperactivity recorded. (Reproduced from Fig. 12 of Maccagnani *et al.* 1966.)

for removal of K^+ from the immediate extraneuronal environment following neuronal activity and hence with the role of the astroglia in maintaining normal neuronal excitability (Orkand *et al.* 1966). The epileptogenic neuron provides an excellent example of the type of problem that is directly relevant to such mechanisms. In this context perhaps the best model is provided by the cardiac glycoside, ouabain (or G-strophanthin), which upon direct intracerebral administration causes severe, prolonged and usually fatal seizures in a variety of mammalian species (Fig. 6) (Ames *et al.* 1965; Cserr 1965; Katzman *et al.* 1965; Maccagnani *et al.* 1966). Ouabain is familiar to biochemists and physiologists as a specific inhibitor of the transport of monovalent cations (Na^+ and K^+) across cell membranes in association with its inhibition of the membrane-bound, Mg-dependent, Na-K-activated ATPase (adenosine triphosphatase), an enzyme which is presumed to mediate the energy transduction required for such transport (Siegel and Albers 1970). The effects of ouabain on a number of aspects of CNS metabolism are summarized in Table V.

TABLE V

EFFECTS OF OUABAIN (10^{-5} M) ON VARIOUS ASPECTS OF CNS METABOLISM

Observations	Control	+ Ouabain[1]
In vitro (cerebral cortex)		
Intracellular K^+ (mM)	119	41
Intracellular Na^+ (mM)	29	96
Mg, Na-K-ATPase		
(mmoles P_i released/g/hr.)	1.52	0[2]
O_2 consumption (μ moles/g/hr.)		
calcium present	64.3	89.4
calcium-free	119.5	96.0
Tissue calcium		
Incubated slices (μ moles/g)	3.6	4.9
Homogenate (μ moles/mg protein)	25.1	35.2
Mitochondria (μ moles/mg protein)	13.35	43.6
In vivo (cerebrum)		
CSF K^+ (mM)		
from choroid plexus	3.3	5.1
during ventriculo-cisternal perfusion	3.2	3.8

[1] All changes from control values are statistically significant at $P < 0.01$ or better.
[2] 50% inhibition occurs at $\sim 5 \times 10^{-7}$ M ouabain.
Data have been taken from Bonting *et al.* (1961, 1962); Ames *et al.* (1965); Cserr (1965); Bourke and Tower (1966b) and Tower (1968).

At inhibitory concentrations (10^{-5}M) of ouabain both *in vitro* and *in vivo* the intracellular concentrations of K^+ are severely depleted and replaced by Na^+ (plus Cl^-). The evidence *in vivo* comes from the studies on choroid plexus by Ames *et al.* (1965) and on brains subjected to ventriculo-cisternal perfusion by Cserr (1965) and Katzman *et al.* (1965). In these studies the perfusates collected from the ouabain-inhibited animals were significantly enriched in K^+, which must have derived from the brain parenchyma. Although it seems reasonable to focus our attention on the outward leakage of intracellular K^+ and the effects of accumulated extracellular K^+ on neuronal excitability, another established effect of ouabain in mobilizing cellular Ca^{++} (Tower 1968; Stahl and Swanson 1969) should not be overlooked. It is this mobilization of tissue-(? membrane-) bound Ca^{++} that results in the selective accumulation of Ca^{++} within mitochondria (Tower 1968; Stahl and Swanson 1969) and the consequent effects on cellular respiratory metabolism (Bourke and Tower 1966b; Tower 1968). Since Ca^{++} stabilizes neural membranes (Shanes 1958), its mobilization therefrom by ouabain could be expected to alter the conformation and hence the permeability and excitability characteristics of the membranes. The electron microscopic observations of Birks (1962) on the morphological changes in neurons of sympathetic ganglia perfused with inhibitory concentrations of cardiac glycoside are of interest in the foregoing context. The visible changes induced by the glycoside could be prevented by use of chloride-free or low-sodium perfusates.

In addition to the example provided by the administration *in vivo* of ouabain, various other types of evidence implicate disturbances of electrolyte (especially K^+) metabolism in seizure states. These observations begin with the classical study by Colfer and Essex (1947) on shifts of Na^+ into and K^+ out of neurons concomitantly with the occurrence of seizure activity. More recently Lewin *et al.* (1969) have reported that in the discharging cortical lesion produced by freezing, the Na-K-ATPase activity is significantly elevated, but it is not clear whether this represents a compensatory increase (on analogy with cholinesterase) (Pope *et al.* 1947; Tower and Elliott 1952b) or an unmasking of latent enzymatic activity as a result of the associated edema and other changes. Fertziger and Ranck (1970) have adduced evidence in favor of accumulation of K^+ in the interstitial spaces surrounding neurons during seizures. And Tower (1965) reported that slices of cerebral cortex from human epileptogenic foci are unable to reaccumulate lost K^+ and extrude excess Na^+ during incubation *in vitro*, in distinct contrast to control slices from non-epileptogenic areas in the human brain.

Glia and seizures

The two lines of investigation that I have considered here, the role of glial cells in buffering the immediate extraneuronal space against excessive external K^+ and the presumptive correlation of epileptogenicity with disturbances of electrolyte (especially K^+) metabolism, converge in the hypothesis proposed by Pollen and Trachtenberg (1970). The studies of these investigators on normal astrocytes of mammalian cerebral cortex complement the earlier data on glia in non-mammalian CNS (Orkand *et al.* 1966) and strengthen the concept of astroglia as a "spatial buffering system" designed to transport excess K^+ away from sites of K^+ release and hence to prevent abnormally increased neuronal excitability. In the epileptogenic focus, Pollen and Trachtenberg (1970) propose that in the commonly associated gliosis the reactive astrocytes may be unable to perform the K^+ buffering function of normal astrocytes and hence would contribute directly to neuronal hyperexcitability (Fig. 7). What is suggested is that at least some forms of epilepsy may be a glial rather than a neuronal disorder.

One additional line of evidence may amplify this concept. Very recently Haber *et al.* (1970) have reported the occurrence of a second type of glutamic decarboxylase (GAD), the enzyme which synthesizes γ-aminobutyric acid (GABA) from glutamic acid. The classical enzyme, designated GAD-I, is restricted in its distribution in the mammalian body to the CNS where it is probably localized primarily in synaptosomes. The GAD-I enzyme is characteristically inhibited by anions and carbonyl reagents. In contrast, the newly-discovered second enzyme GAD-II is widely distributed in many bodily tissues, including blood vessels, and in the CNS is apparently restricted to glial cells. It is characteristically activated by anions and carbonyl reagents (Haber *et al.* 1970). In view of the strong evidence that GABA is an inhibitory transmitter at invertebrate neuromuscular synapses (Kuffler 1960; Kravitz and Potter 1965; Otsuka *et al.* 1966) and at many mammalian central synapses (Obata 1965; Krnjević and Schwartz 1966) the potential involvement of GAD-II and hence of GABA in the proposed glial buffering system is most intriguing. The situation has been depicted schematically in Fig. 7.

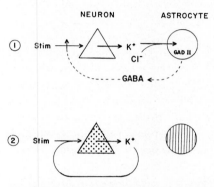

Fig. 7. Schematic depiction of neuron-glia interrelationships, as discussed in the text. *1:* represents for normal cells the "K^+ buffering" action of the astrocyte and the presumed associated release of GABA resulting from activation by Cl^- of GAD-II in the astrocyte. *2:* depicts the lack of occurrence of these events during activity of an epileptogenic neuron because of the unresponsiveness of the fibrous astroglia in the gliotic scar investing the neuron. Adapted from the data reported in: Orkand *et al.* 1966; Bourke 1969 a,b; Haber *et al.* 1970; Pollen and Trachtenberg 1970.

Under normal circumstances, the K^+ released from the neuron as a result of stimulation (or activity) is thought of as entering the adjacent astrocyte by the mediated transport system already postulated (Orkand *et al.* 1966; Bourke 1969a; Trachtenberg and Pollen 1970) accompanied by Cl^- as the anion (Bourke 1969a). Since Cl^- activates the GAD-II of glial cells (Haber *et al.* 1970), an output of GABA could be expected as extra Cl^- entered the astrocyte. Thus, not only would excess K^+ be removed from the immediate extraneuronal environment but any excessive stimulation of the neuron would be modulated by the GABA subsequently released. In contrast the reactive astrocytes in the gliotic area investing epileptogenic neurons would not respond to the K^+ released from the active neuron (Pollen and Trachtenberg 1970), and hence hyperexcitability would ensue or persist.

These concepts add some interesting new dimensions to the problem of epileptogenicity. A critical testing of the hypothesis would seemingly require the isolation and examination of uncontaminated fractions of normal and reactive glia, procedures

References pp. 54–57

which are not now feasible and for which future prospects are not yet very encouraging. There are some other problems especially with reference to the developing nervous system. The neonatal and immature brain tends to be less susceptible to seizures (Purpura 1969) and yet the key elements of the buffering system probably mature at later periods postnatally. There is a late proliferation of glial elements (presumably astrocytes) in both the rat and the kitten (Brizee and Jacobs 1959a, b) that correlates with the late acquisition by kitten cerebral cortex of the propensity to swell upon incubation *in vitro* (Tower and Bourke 1966). Furthermore the classical GABA-synthesizing system is poorly represented in the fetal and neonatal brain and tends to develop in parallel with dendritic maturation (Sisken *et al.* 1961; Berl and Purpura 1963; Baxter 1970). Yet the neonatal brain is apparently sensitive (at least *in vitro*) to ouabain (Table I; Tower 1968). Another consideration at any age is the mechanism(s) by which the astroglia dispose of the excess K^+ (and Cl^-) in order to remain functional as buffering elements. The foregoing exemplify a few of the aspects that require elucidation in terms of the hypothesis propounded.

Envoi

Nevertheless it is both challenging and refreshing to see how rather diverse interests in problems of fluid and electrolyte distribution, cerebral edema, neuronal excitability, glial cell functions, and inhibitory transmitters are now converging to provide us with a new look at some old and perplexing problems. Perhaps these data and concepts will intrigue Herbert Jasper not only because many of them relate to life-long research interests of his but also because it is this sort of convergence of studies and findings that has so often concerned him in his research and teaching. It was with this in mind that this presentation has been prepared as a small but sincere tribute to a valued friend of many years and to a greatly admired colleague.

REFERENCES

ALEU, F. P., KATZMAN, R. and TERRY, R. D. Structure and electrolyte analyses of cerebral edema induced by alkyl tin intoxication. *J. Neuropath. exp. Neurol.*, **1963**, *22*: 403–413.

AMES III, A., HIGASHI, K. and NESBETT, F. B. Effects of P_{CO2}, acetazolamide and ouabain on volume and composition of choroid plexus fluid. *J. Physiol. (Lond.)*, **1965**, *181*: 516–524.

AMES III, A., WRIGHT, R. L., KOWADA, M., THURSTON, J. M. and MAJNO, G. Cerebral ischemia II. The no-reflow phenomenon. *Amer. J. Path.*, **1968**, *52*: 437–453.

BAXTER, C. F. The nature of γ-aminobutyric acid. In A. LAJTHA (Ed.), *Handbook of Neurochemistry*, Vol. 3. Plenum, New York, **1970**: 289–353.

BERL, S. and PURPURA, D. P. Postnatal changes in amino acid content of kitten cerebral cortex. *J. Neurochem.*, **1963**, *10*: 237–240.

BIRKS, R. I. The effects of a cardiac glycoside on subcellular structures within nerve cells and their processes in sympathetic ganglia and skeletal muscle. *Canad. J. Biochem.*, **1962**, *40*: 303–313.

BONTING, S. L., CARAVAGGIO, L. L. and HAWKINS, N. M. Studies on sodium-potassium-activated adenosinetriphosphatase IV. Correlation with cation transport sensitive to cardiac glycosides. *Arch. Biochem.*, **1962**, *98*: 413–419.

BONTING, S. L., SIMON, K. A. and HAWKINS, N. M. Studies on sodium-potassium-activated adenosine triphosphatase I. Quantitative distribution in several tissues of the cat. *Arch. Biochem.*, **1961**, *95*: 416–423.

BOURKE, R. S. Evidence for mediated transport of chloride in cat cerebral cortex *in vitro*. *Exp. Brain Res.*, **1969**a, *8*: 219–231.

BOURKE, R.S. Studies of the development and subsequent reduction of swelling of mammalian cerebral cortex under isosmotic conditions *in vitro*. *Exp. Brain Res.*, **1969**b, *8*: 232–248.

BOURKE, R.S. and TOWER, D.B. Fluid compartmentation and electrolytes of cat cerebral cortex *in vitro* – I. Swelling and solute distribution in mature cerebral cortex. *J. Neurochem.*, **1966**a, *13*: 1071–1097.

BOURKE, R.S. and TOWER, D.B. Fluid compartmentation and electrolytes of cat cerebral cortex *in vitro* – II. Sodium, potassium and chloride of mature cerebral cortex. *J. Neurochem.*, **1966**b, *13*: 1099–1117.

BOURKE, R.S., GABELNICK, H.L. and YOUNG, O. Mediated transport of chloride from blood into cerebrospinal fluid. *Exp. Brain Res.*, **1970**a, *10*: 17–38.

BOURKE, R.S., GREENBERG, E.S. and TOWER, D.B. Variation of cerebral cortex fluid spaces *in vivo* as a function of species brain size. *Amer. J. Physiol.*, **1965**, *208*: 682–692.

BOURKE, R.S., NELSON, K.M., NAUMANN, R.A. and YOUNG, O.M. Studies on the production and subsequent reduction of swelling in primate cerebral cortex under isosmotic conditions *in vivo*. *Exp. Brain Res.*, **1970**b, *10*: 427–446.

BRIGHTMAN, M.W. The distribution within brain of ferritin injected into cerebrospinal fluid compartments. II. Parenchymal distribution. *Amer. J. Anat.*, **1965**, *117*: 193–220.

BRIZEE, K.R. and JACOBS, L.A. Postnatal changes in volumetric and density relationships of neurons in cerebral cortex of cat. *Acta anat. (Basel)*, **1959**a, *38*: 291–303.

BRIZEE, K.R. and JACOBS, L.A. The glia/neuron index in the submolecular layers of the motor cortex of the cat. *Anat. Rec.*, **1959**b, *134*: 97–105.

CHIANG, J., KOWADA, M., AMES III, A., WRIGHT, R.L. and MAJNO, G. Cerebral ischemia III. Vascular changes. *Amer. J. Path.*, **1968**, *52*: 455–476.

CLASEN, R.A., SKY-PECK, H.H., PANDOLFI, S., LAING, I, and HASS, G.M. The chemistry of isolated edema fluid in experimental cerebral injury. In I. KLATZO and F. SEITELBERGER (Eds.), *Brain Edema*. Springer-Verlag, New York, **1967**: 536–553.

COLFER, H.F. and ESSEX, H.E. Distribution of total electrolyte, potassium and sodium in cerebral cortex in relation to experimental convulsions. *Amer. J. Physiol.*, **1947**, *150*: 27–36.

CSERR, H. Potassium exchange between cerebrospinal fluid, plasma and brain. *Amer. J. Physiol.*, **1965**, *209*: 1219–1226.

DAVSON, H. *Physiology of the Ocular and Cerebrospinal Fluid*. Little, Brown, Boston, **1965**: 229.

FARQUHAR, M.G. and HARTMANN, F.G. Neuroglial structure and relationships as revealed by electron microscopy. *J. Neuropath. exp. Neurol.*, **1957**, *16*: 18–39.

FENSTERMACHER, J.D., LI, C-L. and LEVIN, A. Extracellular space of the cerebral cortex of normothermic and hypothermic cats. *Exp. Neurol.*, **1970**, *27*: 101–114.

FERTZIGER, A.P. and RANCK Jr., J.B. Potassium accumulation in interstitial space during epileptiform seizures. *Exp. Neurol.*, **1970**, *26*: 571–585.

FRIEDE, R. Der quantitative Anteil der Glia an der Cortexentwicklung. *Acta anat. (Basel)*, **1954**, *20*: 290–296.

FRIEDMAN, S.B., AUSTEN, W.G., RIESELBACH, R.E., BLOCK, J.B. and RALL, D.P. Effects of hypochloremia on cerebrospinal fluid chloride concentration in a patient with anorexia nervosa and in dogs. *Proc. Soc. exp. Biol. (N.Y.)*, **1963**, *114*: 801–805.

GERSCHENFELD, H.M., WALD, F., ZADUNAISKY, J.A. and DE ROBERTIS, E.D.P. Function of astroglia in the water-ion metabolism of the central nervous system. *Neurology (Minneap.)*, **1959**, *9*: 412–425.

HABER, B., KURIYAMA, K. and ROBERTS, E. L-glutamic acid decarboxylase: a new type in glial cells and human brain gliomas. *Science*, **1970**, *168*: 598.

HAWKINS, A. and OLSZEWSKI, J. Glia/nerve cell index for cortex of the whale. *Science*, **1957**, *126*: 76–77.

KATZMAN, R., GRAZIANI, L., KAPLAN, R. and ESCRIVA, A. Exchange of cerebrospinal fluid potassium with blood and brain. *Arch. Neurol. (Chic.)*, **1965**, *13*: 513–524.

KEESEY, J.C., WALLGREN, H. and McILWAIN, H. The sodium, potassium and chloride of cerebral tissues: maintenance, change on stimulation and subsequent recovery. *Biochem. J.*, **1965**, *95*: 289–300.

KLATZO, I., PIRAUX, A. and LASKOWSKI, E.J. The relationship between edema, blood-brain barrier and tissue elements in a local brain injury. *J. Neuropath. exp. Neurol.*, **1958**, *17*: 548–564.

KLATZO, I., WISNIEWSKI, H. and SMITH, D.E. Observations on the penetration of serum proteins into the central nervous system. *Progr. Brain Res.*, **1965**, *15*: 73–88.

KOCH, A., RANCK JR., J.B. and NEWMAN, B.L. Ionic content of neuroglia. *Exp. Neurol.*, **1962**, *6*: 186–200.

KOROBKIN, R. K., LORENZO, A. V. and CUTLER, R. W. P. Distribution of C^{14}-sucrose and I^{125}-iodide in the central nervous system of the cat after various routes of injection into the cerebrospinal fluid. *J. Pharmacol. exp. Ther.*, **1968**, *164*: 412–420.

KRAVITZ, E. A. and POTTER, D. D. A further study of the distribution of γ-aminobutyric acid between excitatory and inhibitory axons of the lobster. *J. Neurochem.*, **1965**, *12*: 323–328.

KRNJEVIĆ, K. and SCHWARTZ, S. Is γ-aminobutyric acid an inhibitory transmitter? *Nature (Lond.)*, **1966**, *211*: 1372–1374.

KUFFLER, S. W. Excitation and inhibition in single nerve cells. *Harvey Lect. 1958–1959*, **1960**: 176–218.

KUFFLER, S. W. and POTTER, D. D. Glia in the leech central nervous system. Physiological properties and neuron-glia relationship. *J. Neurophysiol.*, **1964**, *27*: 290–320.

KUFFLER, S. W., NICHOLLS, J. G. and ORKAND, R. K. Physiological properties of glial cells in the central nervous system of amphibia. *J. Neurophysiol.*, **1966**, *29*: 768–787.

LEWIN, E., CHARLES, G. and McCRIMMON, A. Discharging cortical lesions produced by freezing: the effect of anticonvulsants on sodium-potassium-activated ATPase, sodium, and potassium in cortex. *Neurology (Minneap.)*, **1969**, *19*: 565–569.

MACCAGNANI, F., BIGNAMI, A. et PALLADINI, G. Etude électroencéphalographique des effets de l'introduction intracranienne d'ouabaïne chez le rat et le cobaye; mise en évidence d'un tracé périodique. *Rev. neurol.*, **1966**, *115*: 211–222.

NICHOLLS, J. G. and KUFFLER, S. W. Extracellular space as a pathway for exchange between blood and neurons in the central nervous system of leech: the ionic composition of glial cells and neurons. *J. Neurophysiol.*, **1964**, *27*: 645–671.

NORRIS, J. W. and PAPPIUS, H. M. Cerebral water and electrolytes. Effects of asphyxia, hypoxia and hypercapnia. *Arch. Neurol. (Chic.)*, **1970**, *23*: 248–258.

OBATA, K. Pharmacological study of postsynaptic inhibition of Deiters' neurones. *Abstr. Commun. 13th Int. Congr. Physiol. Sci. (Tokyo)*, **1965**: 406.

ORKAND, R. K., NICHOLLS, J. G. and KUFFLER, S. W. Effect of nerve impulses on the membrane potential of glial cells in the central nervous system of amphibia. *J. Neurophysiol.*, **1966**, *29*: 788–806.

OTSUKA, M., IVERSEN, L. L., HALL, Z. W. and KRAVITZ, E. A. Release of gamma-aminobutyric acid from inhibitory nerves of lobster. *Proc. Nat. Acad. Sci. (Wash.)*, **1966**, *56*: 1110–1115.

PAPPIUS, H. M. and GULATI, D. R. Water and electrolyte content of cerebral tissues in experimentally induced edema. *Acta neuropath. (Berl.)* **1963**, *2*: 451–460.

POLLEN, D. A. and TRACHTENBERG, M. C. Neuroglia: gliosis and focal epilepsy. *Science*, **1970**, *167*: 1252–1253.

POPE, A., MORRIS, A. A., JASPER, H. ELLIOTT, K. A. C. and PENFIELD, W. Histochemical and action potential studies on epileptogenic areas of cerebral cortex in man and the monkey. *Res. Publ. Ass. nerv. ment. Dis.*, **1947**, *26*: 218–233.

PURPURA, D. P. Stability and seizure susceptibility of immature brain. In H. H. JASPER, A. A. WARD JR. and A. POPE (EDS.), *Basic mechanisms of the epilepsies*. Little, Brown, Boston, **1969**: 481–505.

RALL, D. P., OPPELT, W. W. and PATLACK, C. S. Extracellular space of brain as determined by diffusion of inulin from the ventricular system. *Life Sci.*, **1962**: 43–48.

RANCK JR., J. B. and BeMent, S. L. The specific impedance of the dorsal columns of the cat: an anisotropic medium. *Exp. Neurol.*, **1965**, *11*: 451–462.

REED, D. J. and WOODBURY, D. M. Kinetics of movement of iodide, sucrose, inulin and radio-iodinated albumin in the central nervous system and cerebrospinal fluid of the rat. *J. Physiol. (Lond.)*, **1963**, *169*: 816–850.

SHANES, A. M. Electrochemical aspects of physiological and pharmacological action in excitable cells. *Pharmacol. Rev.*, **1958**, *10*: 59–273.

SIEGEL, G. J. and ALBERS, R. W. Nucleoside triphosphate phosphohydrolases. In A. LAJTHA (ED.), *Handbook of Neurochemistry*, *Vol. 4*. Plenum, New York, **1970**: 13–44.

SISKEN, B., SANO, K. and ROBERTS, E. γ-Aminobutyric acid content and glutamic decarboxylase and γ-aminobutyrate transaminase activities in the optic lobe of the developing chick. *J. biol. Chem.*, **1961**, *236*: 503–507.

STAHL, W. L. and SWANSON, P. D. Uptake of calcium by subcellular fractions isolated from ouabain-treated cerebral tissues. *J. Neurochem.*, **1969**, *16*: 1553–1563.

STEWART-WALLACE, A. M. Biochemical study of cerebral tissue, and changes in cerebral edema. *Brain*, **1939**, *62*: 426–438.

TOWER, D. B. Structural and functional organization of mammalian cerebral cortex: the correlation of neurone density with brain size. Cortical neurone density in the fin whale *(Balaenoptera physalus L.)*, with a note on the cortical neurone density in the Indian elephant. *J. comp. Neurol.*, **1954**, *101*: 19–52.

TOWER, D.B. Problems associated with studies of electrolyte metabolism in normal and epileptogenic cerebral cortex. *Epilepsia (Amst.)*, **1965**, *6*: 183–197.

TOWER, D.B. Distribution of cerebral fluids and electrolytes *in vivo* and *in vitro*. In I. KLATZO and F. SEITELBERGER (EDS.), *Brain edema.* Springer-Verlag. New York, **1967**: 303–332.

TOWER, D.B. Ouabain and the distribution of calcium and magnesium in cerebral tissues *in vitro*. *Exp. Brain Res.*, **1968**, *6*: 273–283.

TOWER, D.B. and BOURKE, R.S. Fluid compartmentation and electrolytes of cat cerebral cortex *in vitro*. III. Ontogenetic and comparative aspects. *J. Neurochem.*, **1966**, *13*: 1119–1137.

TOWER, D.B. and ELLIOTT, K.A.C. Activity of acetylcholine system in cerebral cortex of various unanesthetized mammals. *Amer. J. Physiol.*, **1952a**, *168*: 747–759.

TOWER, D.B. and ELLIOTT, K.A.C. Activity of acetylcholine system in human epileptogenic focus. *J. appl. Physiol.*, **1952b**, *4*: 669–676.

TRACHTENBERG, M.C. and POLLEN, D.A. Neuroglia: biophysical properties and physiological function. *Science*, **1970**, *167*: 1248–1252.

VAN HARREVELD, A. and SCHADÉ, J.P. On the distribution and movements of water and electrolytes in the cerebral cortex. In D.B. TOWER and J.P. SCHADÉ (EDS.), *Structure and function of the cerebral cortex.* Elsevier, Amsterdam, **1960**: 239–254.

VAN HARREVELD, A., CROWELL, J. and MALHOTRA, S.K. A study of extracellular space in central nervous tissue by freeze-substitution. *J. cell Biol.*, **1965**, *25*: 117–137.

VARON, S. and McILWAIN, H. Fluid content and compartments in isolated cerebral tissues. *J. Neurochem.*, **1961**, *8*: 262–275.

WAELSCH, H. An attempt at integration of structure and metabolism in the nervous system. In D.B. TOWER and J.P. SCHADÉ (EDS), *Structure and function of the cerebral cortex.* Elsevier, Amsterdam, **1960**: 313–326.

WANKO, T. and TOWER, D.B. Combined morphological and biochemical studies of incubated slices of cerebral cortex. In M.M. COHEN and R.S. SNIDER (EDS.), *Morphological and biochemical correlates of neural activity.* Hoeber-Harper, New York, **1964**: 75–97.

WOODBURY, D.M. Distribution of nonelectrolytes and electrolytes in brain as affected by alterations in cerebrospinal fluid secretion. In A. LAJTHA and D.H. FORD (EDS.), *Brain-barrier systems.* Elsevier, Amsterdam, **1968**: 297–314.

WOODWARD, D.L., REED, D.J. and WOODBURY, D.M. Extracellular space of rat cerebral cortex. *Amer. J. Physiol.*, **1967**, *212*: 367–370.

Topographical Distribution and Patterns of Unit Activity During Electrically Induced After-Discharge

ROBERT M. CROWELL AND COSIMO AJMONE MARSAN

Branch of Electroencephalography and Clinical Neurophysiology, National Institute of Neurological Diseases and Stroke, National Institutes of Health, Bethesda, Md. 20014 (U.S.A.)

A focal epileptogenic process can be defined as a more or less discrete population of cerebral neurons characterized by an abnormally low threshold of excitability, a susceptibility to large membrane depolarization shifts, and a marked tendency to massive, synchronous activation. This randomly recurring, paroxysmal activation probably reflects the response of the affected neuronal aggregate to minor changes in the normal and, as a rule, subliminal synaptic impingement which originates continuously from various intracerebral structures and the periphery. This abnormal response is generally of relatively brief duration but might occasionally become self-sustained and develop into long lasting phenomena in the form of what we call ictal episodes or seizures.

In the human situation, our understanding of the essence of a focal epileptogenic process is still rather poor. Except for the empirical observation that such a process often develops in proximity to certain lesions or in the course of certain pathological syndromes of the brain (Penfield and Jasper 1954), the mechanisms underlying its formation remain unknown. We are familiar with the numerous and multiform aspects of its peripheral and gross electrographic manifestations, but our knowledge of their pathophysiological substrate is far from complete.

Experimentally, the situation is somewhat better. As a result of the work carried out in different laboratories in the last ten years (see references in Ajmone Marsan 1969) we now possess, at least, a fairly accurate knowledge of the functional behavior of individual elements within the neuronal population artificially affected by an epileptogenic agent, both in "resting" conditions and in the course of their inter-ictal and ictal manifestations.

It should be pointed out, however, that the above definition of a focal epileptic process, which may be accepted as a conceptually valid and useful definition, remains rather vague as to the extent and limits of the involved neuronal population. Indeed, the definition of these parameters presents a difficult problem even in the experimental situation, in which the epileptogenic agent is known and its topographical distribution and site of direct effects can be, at least partially, controlled; the same problem becomes practically insoluble in the much less favorable, human situation. Among the factors which contribute to this difficulty is one of the most characteristic properties of the epileptogenic process itself; namely, its marked tendency to spread and to involve in its activity wider and wider regions of the central nervous system, including distant neuronal populations which are "normal" and which, in any case, could reasonably be considered as not directly affected by the epileptogenic agent. This situation creates a number of both practical and basic problems. It not only complicates or prevents the definition of the exact functional delimitation of a focal epileptogenic process, but also contributes to the complexities of diagnosis and to a considerable share of surgical-therapeutic failures in the clinical field. Furthermore, as a result of their invasion by, and possible active involvement in epileptiform activation, the functional properties of an undetermined number of normal neuronal aggregates are seriously disrupted during ictal episodes and probably impaired in the inter-ictal periods. Finally, there is also a theoretical possibility, apparently supported by some suggestive experimental evidence (Morrell 1959; Wilder and Morrell 1967) that certain neuronal populations preferentially subjected to this abnormal activation, might become capable of autonomous epileptic behavior independently from, or even in the absence of, the primary epileptogenic process.

Our continous interest in the basic mechanism of seizure activity has been recently focused on these general aspects. Specifically, we have tried to analyze the neuronal behavior in parts of the cerebral cortex which are not directly affected by the epileptogenic agent and yet appear to participate in its effects. Indeed, by superficial observation and without the use of direct-coupled (DC) amplifiers, the gross electrographic manifestations of these remote regions may often look quite similar to those of the directly affected populations. The behavior of these distant neurons during the paroxysmal inter-ictal, short-lasting events has been investigated in previous works (Ajmone Marsan 1963; Crowell 1970). Here we plan to report our results in relation to the longer duration ictal episodes. In this series of experiments a comparison has been made of the changes in the activity of the same neuron in the course of electrical after-discharges (AD) of various origin. Special attention has been paid to the relationship of the neuronal location to the site of the repetitive electrical stimulation in determining unit activity patterns during these ictal events. In particular, a deliberate search for "surround inhibition" (Prince and Wilder 1967; Dichter and Spencer 1969a) in relation to ictal discharge has been carried out. In addition, the influence of pentobarbital anesthesia upon unit discharge patterns during AD induced by contralateral stimulation has been assessed.

METHODS

Acute experiments were performed in forty-three cats. Surgical procedures were carried out during the administration of ether anesthesia. After tracheal incannulation, ether was discontinued and, after administration of D-tubocurarine (1.5 mg/kg i.v.), artificial ventilation was begun. A bilateral frontal craniectomy was performed with a wide cortical exposure on one side and a small (4–5 mm diameter) exposure of the anterior sigmoid gyrus on the opposite side. In order to limit cortical pulsations, bilateral pneumothorax and axial elevation were employed in most experiments. All pressure points and wound edges were carefully infiltrated with 2% Novocaine [R] at regular intervals.

The experimental situation is shown schematically in Fig. 1. For convenience of description, the anterior sigmoid gyrus penetrated by the micro-pipette is termed "ipsi" and that of the contralateral hemisphere is called "contra". Ag-AgCl electrodes monitored electrocorticographic (ECoG) activity of each of these two gyri (clamps fixed to the lateral wound edges serving as referential electrodes). The "ipsi" ECoG electrode was located about 1 mm medial to the micro-pipette. Micro-pipettes filled with 2M potassium citrate and having tip resistances in saline of 10–50 MΩ were used to record neuronal activity in "ipsi" anterior sigmoid gyrus, about 6–9 mm lateral to the midline. A saline electrode attached to the occipital wound edge served as grounded reference. Pairs of stainless steel electrodes (tip separation about 1.0 mm) were used for repetitive electrical stimulation to elicit ADs. The "ipsi" stimulating pair straddled the micro-pipette for "direct" stimulation (27 animals) or lay 2–4 mm lateral to the micro-pipette for "local" stimulation (9 animals). The "contra" electrode pair was usually located at the contralateral point roughly homotopic to the point of micro-electrode penetration. In 5 experiments, a roving pair of stimulating electrodes was used to survey a large number of points in the "contra" pericruciate cortex. Trains of pulses (1–3 msec, 20–100/sec, 10–50 V) were used to elicit ADs.

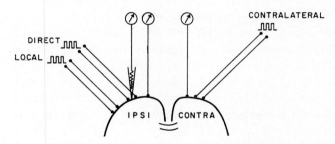

Fig. 1. Schematic representation of the experimental conditions. The anterior sigmoid gyri are labelled IPSI on the side sampled by the micro-electrode and CONTRA on the contralateral hemisphere. Surface (referential) electrodes record electrocorticographic (ECoG) activity from both hemispheres. Three pairs of electrodes were used for repetitive electrical stimulation: one straddling the micro-electrode for *direct* stimulation, the other placed 2–4 mm away from the micro-pipette for *local* stimulation and the pair placed on the opposite hemisphere, roughly homotopic to the micro-electrode, for *contralateral* stimulation.

In eight cats in which only gross surface recording was employed, section of the corpus callosum was carried out according to the method described by Magni *et al.* (1960).

ECoGs were led through Tektronix Model 122 amplifiers (time constant: 1 sec), and micro-electrode activity was led DC through a Bak unity gain amplifier and a Quan-Tech Model 201B decade amplifier. All signals were displayed on a Tektronix model 535 4-beam cathode ray oscilloscope. Photographs on moving film were made with a Grass Kymograph camera.

References pp. 72–73

A hydraulic micro-manipulator was used to advance the micro-electrode. After the latter was brought into contact with the surface of the "ipsi" cortex, a 3% agar solution at 37°C was applied to this area and allowed to solidify. Experiments were started at least 4 h after the discontinuation of ether anesthesia.

RESULTS

Extracellular records were obtained from 158 units. Intracellular records were derived from 11 neurons which lacked obvious signs of damage and maintained resting membrane potentials of 35–60 mV (supplementary data from 8 neurons with similar resting membrane potentials, but with signs of injury, were also utilized). Data were also available from 21 neurons which showed post-synaptic potentials and spike amplitudes of 15 mV or more ("quasi-intracellular" records).

A. *Effects on neuronal firing in the course of ADs resulting from direct, local, and contralateral stimulation.* Unit behavior during AD was classified according to the following criteria: "Synchronous" (SYNCH) firing refers to a temporal association of spike discharges with rhythmic wave forms of the AD in the ipsilateral ECoG. "Activation" refers to an appreciable increase in discharge frequency (↑) or to a rapid (over 30/sec) cellular firing (↑ ↑). "Suppression" (↓) refers to a decrease in discharge frequency, or to an arrest in spike firing. Lack of any appreciable alteration in the spike firing rate during AD was classified as "no change" (NC).

Each of these patterns was observed, although with different incidence, in the course of ADs elicited from the three stimulation sites. Examples of rather unusual unit behavior are shown in Fig. 2 (suppression of unit activity during an AD induced by direct ipsilateral stimulation), Fig. 3 (synchronization of unit activity during an AD induced by contralateral stimulation) and Fig. 4 (marked activation with AD from contralateral stimulation). An example of more common findings, *i.e.*, suppression of spikes during contralaterly induced AD, is shown in Fig. 5.

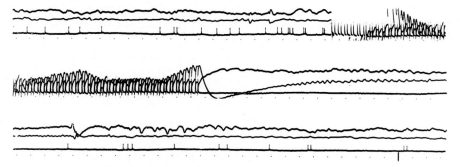

Fig. 2. Suppression of unit activity during AD following direct ipsilateral stimulation. In this and succeeding figures, the top trace is ECoG ipsilateral to the micro-electrode, the middle trace is ECoG contralateral thereto, and the bottom trace is the micro-electrode record. Negativity is up in ECoG tracings and down in the micro-electrode tracing. Note cessation of firing and mild hyperpolarization during AD. Calibration for intracellular recording: 60 mV. Time: 200 msec.

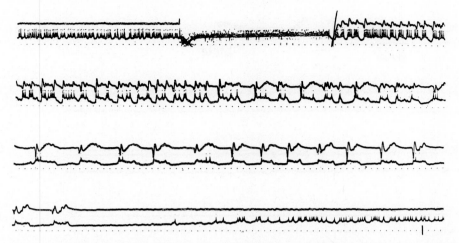

Fig. 3. Synchronized activity in a unit during AD following contralateral stimulation. ECoG trace from cortex contralateral to micro-electrode is absent. Note synchronization of the neuronal post-synaptic potentials with the surface ECoG, especially during the clonic phase. See Fig. 2 for further explanations. Calibration for intracellular record: 40 mV. Time: 200 msec.

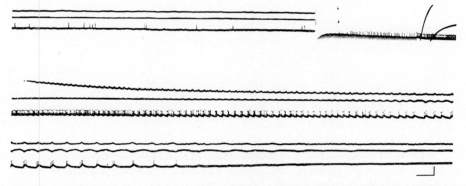

Fig. 4. Marked activation in a unit during AD following contralateral stimulation. After repetitive stimulation, an AD arises and is projected to the hemisphere of micro-electrode penetration. Note the rapid neuronal discharge during the tonic phase, synchronous burst discharge during the clonic phase, and long-lasting post-ictal unit suppression. See Fig. 2 for further explanations. Calibration for extracellular record: 10 mV. Time marker: 1 sec.

Since any given unit tended to behave consistently during successive ADs of identical origin (provided the ictal episodes were of comparable duration[1]), it was possible to classify neurons with regard to typical behavior pattern in relation to the various types

[1] It is conceivable that different effects subsequent to ipsilateral and contralateral repetitive stimulation could merely be the expression of differences in the "intensities" of ADs induced locally and projected contralaterally. It is difficult to quantify AD "intensity", since both amplitude of individual waves and intrinsic AD frequency tend to vary through the different stages of any given AD. As a compromise, the total AD duration is commonly used as an indirect measure of the AD "intensity". In these experiments, the average duration of ipsilaterally-evoked AD (direct and local) was 33.5 sec and the average duration of contralaterally evoked (projected) AD was 42.9 sec.

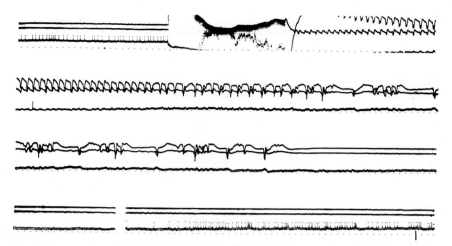

Fig. 5. Suppression of activity in a unit during AD following contralateral stimulation. Note cessation of unit firing during AD which appears prominently in both ECoG records. Single full-sized spike in line 2 suggests that cathodal block is not present. Unit remains silent post-ictally (line 3 and first part of 4). See Fig. 2 for further explanations. Calibration for quasi-intracellular record: 20 mV. Time: 200 msec.

TABLE I

UNIT ACTIVITY DURING ADS OF DIFFERENT ORIGIN

AD origin	Unit Behavior Pattern					
	↑	Synch	↑ ↑	↓	NC	Totals (%)
Direct	14 (18.9)	28 (37.9)	22 (29.7)	7 (9.4)	3 (4.1)	74 (100.0)
Local	18 (13.2)	33 (24.3)	8 (5.9)	37 (27.2)	40 (29.4)	136 (100.0)
Contralateral	24 (12.6)	58 (30.5)	5 (2.6)	40 (21.1)	63 (33.2)	190 (100.0)

of AD (*i.e.*, ictal events produced by direct, local, or contralateral stimulation). The results of this analysis are presented in Table I. The incidence of the various response patterns during directly induced AD was rather different from that of response patterns during locally induced AD and contralaterally induced AD, whereas for these last two the distribution of response patterns was rather similar. Excitatory effects (activation, synchronization and marked activation taken together) were predominant during directly induced AD (86.5%) and common during both locally induced AD (43.4%) and contralaterally induced AD (45.7%). Marked activation, on the other hand, was relatively common during directly induced AD (29.7%) but rare in the other two groups. Suppression and lack of effect were rare during directly evoked AD but relatively common during locally or contralaterally induced ADs.

The activity of 83 neurons was examined during both directly and contralaterally evoked AD, and the behavior of 87 neurons was studied during both locally and contralaterally induced ADs. (No records from any unit were obtained during both directly and locally evoked AD.) These data were utilized to determine whether individual units tended to respond similarly or differently during ADs of different origin. A given unit tended to behave similarly during locally and contralaterally produced

AD, especially when the effects consisted of suppression or were absent. When the effects of directly and contralaterally induced AD were tested on the same unit elements, response patterns were different in some units (see, *e.g.*, Fig. 6) and similar in other units. The latter situation was particularly common when the pattern consisted of synchronization.

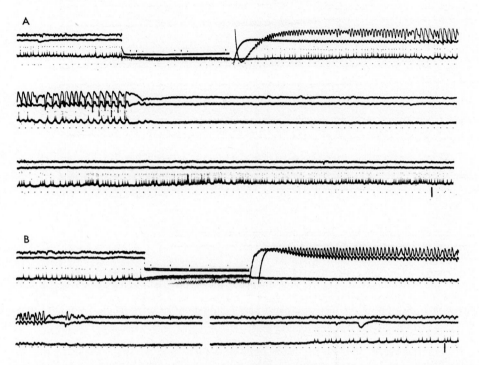

Fig. 6. Different firing patterns in the same neuron during ADs of different origins. *A:* synchronized unit activity during AD following direct ipsilateral stimulation. *B:* suppression of unit activity and hyperpolarization during AD following contralateral stimulation. Note long-lasting post-ictal cessation of firing and hyperpolarization in both *A* and *B*. See Fig. 2 for further explanations. Calibrations for intracellular records: 40 mV. Time: 200 msec.

B. *Changes in membrane potential during ADs induced by direct, local and contralateral stimulation.* The limited number of available intracellular records was surveyed for evidence of sustained membrane depolarization in relation to various ADs. Of 3 neurons in which a record was obtained during directly evoked AD, mild depolarization (3–5 mV) was seen in one, and marked depolarization with spike inactivation was seen in two. Of 7 neurons studied during locally induced AD, moderate depolarization was seen in 4 and marked depolarization with spike inactivation in 3. In 11 neurons whose activity was recorded during contralaterally produced AD, mild membrane depolarization was common, but marked membrane depolarization and spike inactivation never occurred.

A reversible diminution of spike amplitude in extracellular records during AD has been interpreted as indirect evidence of sustained membrane depolarization (Gerin

1960). In those units which showed spike activation, synchronization, or marked activation, spike amplitude decrease of 50% or more (see Fig. 7) was found to be common (42.5%) during direct AD, relatively uncommon (22.2%) during local AD, and rare (6.9%) during contralateral AD.

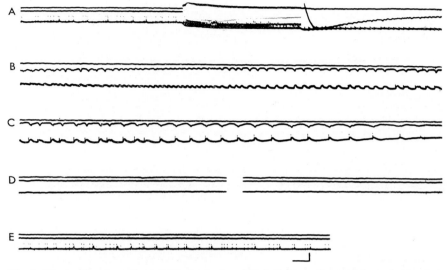

Fig. 7. Diminution in spike amplitude during AD following direct ipsilateral stimulation. Note extreme attenuation of spikes during AD in *A*, disappearance of spikes in *B*, and gradual reappearance of spikes in *B* and *C*. Post-ictal suppression of unit firing occurs in *D*. Spikes recover at their original amplitude in *E*. See Fig. 2 for further explanations. Calibration for extracellular record: 15 mV. Time marker: 1 sec.

C. *ADs elicited from "homotopic" and non-homotopic points.* In 5 experiments, a number of points contralateral to the micro-electrode were stimulated to produce ADs. The activity of 31 units was recorded during ADs elicited from two or more contralateral points. The effects on such units (when present) were classified as excitation or suppression. In comparing the responses of any given unit during ADs of varied contralateral origin, the cell was scored as "consistent" or "inconsistent". About half of the units were inconsistent, but only inasmuch as they would display either excitation and no effect, or suppression and no effect. No unit showed excitation during one AD and suppression in the course of another AD when ADs were induced by stimulation of different points in the contralateral cortex.

D. *"Silent" cells and AD.* Suitable intracellular records were obtained from 10 "silent" cells (see Sugaya *et al.* 1964; Karahashi and Goldring 1966). These elements showed stable resting membrane potentials of 50–90 mV, and stable tracings were secured for 2–10 min. In 4 cells, prominent depolarization (up to 20 mV) was observed in relation to directly induced AD (Fig. 8), while in the remaining cells there was no appreciable depolarization during such ipsilateral epileptogenesis. In all 10 cells, no change in resting membrane potential was recorded in relation to contralaterally evoked AD. Many silent cells (as in the case of that of Fig. 8) showed low-voltage,

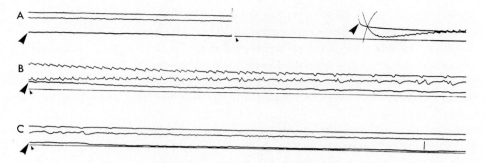

Fig. 8. Depolarization of "silent cell" during AD following direct ipsilateral stimulation. Bottom trace in each line indicates initial resting membrane potential (small arrows). In *A* after repetitive stimulation, top ECoG trace (ipsilateral to stimulation) goes off screen, and intracellular trace (large arrow) shows depolarization of about 25 mV. In *B*, during bilateral seizure activity, intracellular trace (large arrow) shows gradual repolarization and small wave forms in synchrony with ECoG wave forms. In *C* after the end of seizure activity intracellular trace (large arrow) shows almost total repolarization. (Immediately after the illustrated AD, the micro-electrode was withdrawn to an extracellular position; under these conditions AD was associated with no significant change in DC potential.) See Fig. 2 for further explanations. Calibration for intracellular record: 20 mV. Time scale as in Fig. 7.

rhythmical depolarization waves in relation to the surface AD (either local or projected), regardless of whether the sustained depolarization was present or absent.

E. *Effect of callosal section on projected AD.* In all intact preparations, ECoG evidence of AD was present contralateral to the site of repetitive stimulation. In ten of the twelve preparations in which the corpus callosum was sectioned, such a procedure abolished projected discharge. In the other two preparations, in which projected rhythmical activation had persisted in a somewhat attenuated form in the contralateral homologous cortex, autopsy revealed incomplete section of the corpus callosum.

F. *Effects of sodium pentobarbital on projected discharge.* Data from the present study obtained in preparations under D-tubocurarine/Novocaine [R] were compared with those previously obtained (Crowell 1970) in animals maintained on barbiturate anesthesia. The incidence of cells with various behavior patterns during contralaterally induced AD under local anesthesia is shown in Table II. Each possible pattern of activity was noted in the two situations. Under local anesthesia, an excitatory response (activation, synchronization or marked activation) occurred in about half. By contrast, under barbiturate anesthesia, suppression was observed in about half, and excitatory responses occurred in only about one-third of the cells.

TABLE II

UNIT ACTIVITY DURING AD OF CONTRALATERAL ORIGIN DURING LOCAL ANESTHESIA AND DURING BARBITURATE ANESTHESIA

Anesthesia	↑	SYNCH	↑↑	↓	NC	Total
Local anesthesia[1]	24 (12.6%)	58 (30.5%)	5 (2.6%)	40 (21.1%)	63 (33.2%)	190
Barbiturate anesthesia[2]	20 (9.7%)	36 (17.5%)	6 (2.9%)	106 (51.7%)	37 (18.0%)	205

[1] D-tubocurarine, 1.5 mg/kg i.v., and Novocaine [R].
[2] From Crowell (1970); sodium pentobarbital, 35 mg/kg i.p. for fifteen cats, sodium methohexital, 25 mg/kg i.m. for eighteen cats.

G. *Post-ictal phenomena*. In 37 of 43 experiments, ECoG data showed a decrease in surface-recorded wave amplitude ipsilateral to AD origin during the immediate post-ictal period. The effect was most pronounced during the first 10–30 sec post-ictally, but could last up to 3 min. Post-ictal depression was rarely noted contralateral to the origin of AD even though the projected ECoG discharges had been well developed. In the rare instances in which some depression was observed, this followed an AD of remarkably long duration.

Unit data were surveyed for activation, suppression, or lack of effects during the post-ictal period (see examples in Fig. 3–7). As shown in Table III, post-ictal suppression was very common after direct AD, but was noted in less than half of the units after local and contralateral AD. In addition, suppression effects after direct AD tended to be longer lasting than after local or contralateral AD (Table IV). Facilitatory effects were rarely observed. In the few neurons in which intracellular records were obtained, there was little or no evidence for membrane hyperpolarization in coincidence with their post-ictal functional silence (see exception in Fig. 6, *B*); this was the case for all three types of AD.

TABLE III

POST-ICTAL UNIT ACTIVITY IN RELATION TO ADS OF DIFFERENT ORIGINS

AD origin	Unit Activity			Totals
	↑	↓	NC	
Direct	0	43 (78.2)	12 (21.8)	55 (100.0%)
Local	4 (2.9)	68 (48.9)	67 (48.2)	139 (100.0%)
Contralateral	8 (4.1)	91 (46.2)	98 (49.7)	197 (100.0%)

TABLE IV

DURATION OF SUPPRESSION OF POST-ICTAL UNIT ACTIVITY DURING ADS OF DIFFERENT ORIGINS

AD origin	Duration of Suppression (seconds)				Totals
	1–10	11–50	51–100	101–200	
Direct	3 (7.0%)	20 (46.5%)	11 (25.6%)	9 (20.9%)	43 (100.0%)
Local	27 (39.7%)	33 (48.5%)	8 (11.8%)		68 (100.0%)
Contralateral	49 (53.8%)	36 (39.6%)	5 (5.5%)	1 (1.1%)	91 (100.0%)

DISCUSSION

By utilizing a well known phenomenon, thoroughly investigated by Adrian (1939), Moruzzi (1939), Rosenblueth and Cannon (1941–42), Bonnet and Bremer (1956) and many others, the present experiments have reproduced a reasonably good example of the situation to which we referred in the introduction; namely, a focal area of epileptiform activation which is, however, ill-defined and rather extensive, in spite of the relatively discrete application of the epileptogenic agent (represented here by the repetitive electrical stimulation) and of the obviously focal onset of the process. On the basis of gross surface A.C. recording, the various morphological features of this activity appear rather similar throughout the extent of the involved regions. Our findings have also shown, however, that in the course of such ictal episodes, there is a difference in the preferential patterns of behavior of different neuronal aggregates at various distances from the original site of action of the epileptogenic agent, or in the pattern of the same neuronal populations, for different locations of the epileptogenic stimulus. Directly induced AD (*i.e.*, AD induced by stimulating electrodes which straddle the micro-pipette) was predominantly associated with excitatory effects; profound activation with sustained membrane depolarization and spike inactivation were common (see also Sawa *et al.* 1963, 1968; Sugaya *et al.* 1964) and suppression was rare. ADs induced both by local (*i.e.*, ipsilateral but 2–4 mm distant) or contralateral stimulation were associated with either activation or suppression of unit activity, but profound activation and sustained depolarization were uncommon. Unit behavior patterns during directly evoked AD were clearly different from those observed in the course of locally or contralaterally induced ADs.

In the course of inter-ictal discharges of penicillin-induced foci, in motor cortex (Prince and Wilder 1967) or hippocampus (Dichter and Spencer 1969a, b), neurons within the focus show mainly excitatory phenomena while neurons 3–8 mm away have been reported to show predominantly inhibitory phenomena. This "surround inhibition" was less definite in the present experiments in which the ictal activity in nearby ipsilateral and in contralateral areas appeared to be heterogeneous and somewhat more similar to that described by Dichter and Spencer (1969a) in "transitional" regions. The predominance of mixed effects and the scarcity of prominent inhibitory phenomena in these areas may be due to a relative failure of surround inhibition during ictal epileptogenesis (see Dichter and Spencer 1969b).

The differences between the preferential patterns of activity of the neurons situated at the center of the focus and of those at its periphery or at a distance from it, were not clear-cut enough for the practical purpose of outlining the limits of the focus itself, but were sufficient to permit an identification of neuronal populations which are primarily responsible for the epileptogenic process and of those secondarily involved by it. In the latter one finds a relatively large contingent of elements (about one-third) which do not seem to participate in the epileptiform activity, in contrast with a more than 95% participation by the neurons at the center of the focus. Of the units secondarily affected by the epileptogenic process, inhibition of their activity was about four times as common, and excitatory phenomena, when present, were of rather moderate entity. The different degree of intensity of the latter phenomena in the two populations of neurons was particularly interesting. One would seldom observe the intense excitation characterizing the behavior of neurons at the center of the focus, and even when the unit displayed the rhythmical firing of spikes in synchrony with the wave pattern of the ictal episode, the corresponding changes in membrane potential were limited to moderate depolarizing oscillations arising from its resting level (see, however, Sawa *et al.* 1968; Mori 1969). The membrane of the individual elements directly affected by the epileptogenic agent, on the other hand, would show consistently a steady and rather marked depolarization: the rhythmical oscillations developed when the membrane

References pp. 72–73

potential had decreased to a critical level, their frequency varied in relation with minor changes in this level and they would persist as long as such level was maintained. This could be considered as one of the main differences in the mechanisms which are at the basis of the ictal phenomena in the two groups of neurons. More specifically, the typical ictal patterns would be the consequence of an excessive membrane depolarization induced by the epileptogenic stimulus on a relatively limited number of elements which are in the immediate range of its sphere of action. The changes in the elements of surrounding or distant populations may be absent or, if present, merely reflect their synaptic organization and relationship with the primarily affected neurons and correspond to post-synaptic phenomena (either excitatory or inhibitory) generated by the output of the latter. In spite of the obviously unphysiological nature of this output its synaptic drives do not seem to differ substantially from those which are generated under "physiological" conditions (see also Asanuma and Okuda 1962; Krnjevic *et al.* 1966).

Both excitation and inhibition have been reported in regions at a distance from the site of origin of the AD, the nature of the observed effects apparently depending upon the location of stimulation and of unit recording (Yamamoto 1963; Ionescu *et al.* 1967; Yokota and MacLean 1968). The failure to find, in the present study, a contralateral focus of *intense* excitatory activity during AD could simply indicate an overlooking of the very discrete homotopic focus (Asanuma and Okuda 1962). This interpretation appears unlikely in view of the negative results in the five preparations in which roving stimulating electrodes were employed. Differences in type and depth of anesthesia could also account for some of the discrepancies between this study and that of Asanuma and Okuda. More probably, however, the relatively diffuse nature of the phenomena induced by repetitive stimulation and associated with the subsequent AD, could have resulted in widespread, overlapping inhibitory effects which might then overwhelm a focus of projected excitation.

"*Silent*" cells during AD

This study has confirmed that "silent" cells within a focus of AD may display profound depolarization (Sugaya *et al.* 1964; Karahashi and Goldring 1966). Similar events were not observed in a small number of "silent" cells impaled contralateral to the site of stimulation. It is of interest that a contrast between center and (contralateral) surround during AD can be noted even in relation to silent cell activity. The observed changes in silent cell membrane potentials may be related to the ictal DC shift which has been reported to be negative within the focus and predominantly positive contralateral thereto (Gumnit and Takahashi 1965).

Barbiturates and AD

The present results suggest one of the possible neuronal mechanisms which might be involved in the anti-epileptic effects of barbiturates. During local anesthesia, activation is the characteristic response of units contralateral to the site of origin of AD, whereas during barbiturate anesthesia, suppression is the commonest response. Thus, as suggested by Mori (1969), barbiturates appear to diminish excitatory drives and to enhance inhibitory actions upon contralateral neurons in relation to AD. This suppressor action may be a counterpart at the neuronal level to suppression by barbiturate of projected paroxysmal discharge at the ECoG level (Morrell and Baker 1961). The suppression effects observed in the present study may be related to enhancement of inhibitory effects reported by others in a variety of non-epileptic preparations (Marshall 1941; Purpura and Cohen 1962; Poggio and Mountcastle 1963; Andersen *et al.* 1964; Crawford and Curtis 1966; Crawford 1969). In the few intracellular records reported here pronounced hyperpolarization of the neuronal membrane was not observed in neurons contralateral to AD after systemic administration of barbiturate. This suggests the possibility of a pre-synaptic mechanism (see Eccles 1962; Sugaya *et al.* 1964). Whatever the intimate mechanism of action of barbiturates, the present results suggest the need for a certain caution in interpreting data on projected epileptiform discharge in the presence of even light barbiturate anesthesia.

Post-ictal phenomena

Post-ictal depression of ECoG activity was commonly observed at the end of an ictal episode recorded at the site of cortical stimulation, but less commonly after ADs projected to homologous contralateral cortex. Neuronal populations in close proximity to the site of origin of the ictal activity showed long lasting suppression of their firing at the end of the paroxysmal episode whereas fewer units within the region of a projected AD showed post-ictal suppression, even when there was evidence of their participation in the AD itself. This observation represents an additional differential feature in the behavior of neuronal populations characterized by different topographical relationships with the primary epileptogenic stimulus. It may be that antecedent events such as direct effects of this stimulus, marked activation of neuronal populations, or massive depolarization of neuronal membranes are involved in the genesis of subsequent post-ictal depression. Events occurring at the membrane level simultaneous with post-ictal depression remain obscure. Membrane hyperpolarization has only occasionally been observed in neurons during post-ictal depression (Matsumoto and Ajmone Marsan 1964; Sugaya *et al.* 1964) and was uncommon in the present study. Pre-synaptic inhibition, post-synaptic inhibition, neuronal inactivation (Phillips 1958), metabolic "exhaustion" (Dusser de Barenne and McCulloch 1939) or a combination of these could explain the observed results.

SUMMARY

1. Micro-electrode penetrations in the anterior sigmoid gyrus were carried out in forty-three locally anesthetized cats; 158 extracellular, 11 uninjured intracellular, and 21 "quasi-intracellular" records were obtained. Unit behavior was studied during after-discharge (AD) induced by direct, local (2–4 mm distant) or contralateral repetitive electrical stimulation.

2. During ADs, unit spikes showed various degrees of activation, synchronization with ECoG rhythmical waves, suppression, or no change in their firing pattern. Excitatory effects were predominant during directly induced AD and common during

References pp. 72–73

both locally or contralaterally induced AD. Marked activation was rare in the latter two types of AD. Suppression and lack of effect were rare during directly evoked AD but relatively common during locally or contralaterally induced ADs.

3. In the small number of intracellular records, marked depolarization with spike inactivation was observed during AD after ipsilateral stimulation, but never during AD subsequent to contralateral stimulation.

4. No unit showed excitation during one AD and suppression during another AD when ADs were induced by stimulation of different points in contralateral cortex.

5. Intracellular records were also obtained from 10 "silent" cells. Four of these showed prominent depolarization during directly induced AD. None showed any change in resting membrane potential during contralaterally induced AD.

6. A complete callosal section abolished ECoG evidence of projected discharge in all preparations so treated.

7. Data from the present study (local anesthesia) were compared to those from a previous study in which barbiturate anesthesia was employed. Under local anesthesia, an excitatory effect was seen in about half the units during contralaterally induced AD. In the same situation under barbiturate anesthesia, suppression occurred in about half of the units, and excitatory effects were observed in about one-third.

8. ECoG evidence of post-ictal depression occurred very commonly in cortex ipsilateral to stimulation, but only rarely in cortex contralateral to stimulation. Evidence of post-ictal suppression at the unitary level was more common and of longer duration after directly induced AD than after locally or contralaterally induced ADs.

ACKNOWLEDGEMENTS

The authors are indebted to Mrs. D. Yarrow, Mr. J. Jones and Mr. A. Ziminsky for secretarial and technical assistance.

REFERENCES

ADRIAN, E. D. The localization of activity in the brain. *Proc. roy. Soc. London*, **1939**, *B126*: 433–449.
AJMONE MARSAN, C. Unitary analysis of "projected" epileptiform discharges. *Electroenceph. clin. Neurophysiol.*, **1963**, *15*: 197–208.
AJMONE MARSAN, C. Acute effects of topical epileptogenic agents. In H. H. JASPER, A. A WARD JR., and A. POPE (EDS.), *Basic mechanisms of the epilepsies*. Little, Brown, Boston, Mass., **1969**: 299–319.
ANDERSEN, P., ECCLES, J. C. and SEARS, T. A. The ventro-basal complex of the thalamus: types of cells, their responses and their functional organization. *J. Physiol. (Lond.)*, **1964**, *174*: 370–399.
ASANUMA, H. and OKUDA, O. Effects of transcallosal volleys on pyramidal tract cell activity of cat. *J. Neurophysiol.*, **1962**, *25*: 198–208.
BONNET, V. et BREMER, F. Analyse des modifications préconvulsives de la réaction de l'écorce cérébrale à un stimulus direct répété. *J. Physiol. (Paris)*, **1956**, *48*: 399–403.
CRAWFORD, J. M. Effects of convulsant barbiturates on cortical neurons. *Brain Res.*, **1969**, *12*: 485–489.
CRAWFORD, J. M. and CURTIS, D. R. Pharmacological studies on feline Betz cells. *J. Physiol. (Lond.)*, **1966**, *186*: 121–138.

CROWELL, R.M. Distant effects of a focal epileptogenic process. *Brain Res.*, **1970**, *18*:137–154.

DICHTER, M. and SPENCER, W.A. Penicillin-induced inter-ictal discharges from the cat hippocampus. I. Characteristics and topographical features. *J. Neurophysiol.*, **1969**a, *32*: 649–662.

DICHTER, M. and SPENCER, W.A. Penicillin-induced inter-ictal discharges from the cat hippocampus. II. Mechanisms underlying origin and restriction. *J. Neurophysiol.*, **1969**b, *32*: 663–687.

DUSSER DE BARENNE, J.G. and McCULLOCH, W.S. Factors for facilitation and extinction in the central nervous system. *J. Neurophysiol.*, **1939**, *2*: 319–355.

ECCLES, J.C. Spinal neurons: synaptic connections in relation to chemical transmitters and pharmacological responses. In *Proceedings of the First International Pharmacological Meeting*. Pergamon, New York, **1962**, 172p.

GERIN, P. Microelectrode investigations on the mechanisms of the electrically induced epileptiform seizure ("afterdischarge"). *Arch. ital. Biol.*, **1960**, *98*: 21–40.

GUMNIT, R.J. and TAKAHASHI, T. Changes in direct current activity during experimental focal seizures. *Electroenceph. clin. Neurophysiol.*, **1965**, *19*: 63–74.

IONESCU, D.A., SOBIRESCU, N. und VOICULESCU, V. Mikroelektroden-Untersuchung der neocorticalen paroxysmalen Vorgänge nach Hippocampus-Reiz bei der Katze. *Arch. Psychiat. Nervenkr.*, **1967**, *210*: 263–273.

KARAHASHI, Y. and GOLDRING, S. Intracellular potentials from "idle" cells in cerebral cortex of cat. *Electroenceph. clin. Neurophysiol.*, **1966**, *20*: 600–607.

KRNJEVIC, K., RANDIC, M. and STRAUGHAN, D.W. An inhibitory process in the cerebral cortex. *J. Physiol. (Lond.)*, **1966**, *184*: 16–48.

MAGNI, F., MELZACK, R. and SMITH, L.J. A stereotaxic method for sectioning the corpus callosum of the cat. *Electroenceph. clin. Neurophysiol.*, **1960**, *12*: 517–518.

MARSHALL, W.H. Observations on subcortical somatic sensory mechanisms of cats under Nembutal anesthesia. *J. Neurophysiol.*, **1941**, *4*: 25–43.

MATSUMOTO, H. and AJMONE MARSAN, C. Cortical cellular phenomena in experimental epilepsy: ictal manifestations. *Exp. Neurol.*, **1964**, *9*: 305–326.

MORI, K. Single unit study of the projected after-discharge in neocortex. *Acta med. Univ. Kyoto*, **1969**, *40*: 194–203.

MORRELL, F. Secondary epileptogenic lesions. *Epilepsia (Amst.)*, **1959**, *1*: 538–560.

MORRELL, F. and BAKER, L. Effects of drugs on secondary epileptogenic lesions. *Neurology (Minneap.)*, **1961**, *11*: 651–664.

MORUZZI, G. Contribution à l'électrophysiologie du cortex moteur: facilitation, afterdischarge et épilepsie corticale. *Arch. int. Physiol.*, **1939**, *49*: 33–100.

PENFIELD, W. and JASPER, H. *Epilepsy and the functional anatomy of the human brain*. Little, Brown, Boston, **1954**: 896p.

PHILLIPS, C.G. Actions of antidromic pyramidal volleys on single Betz cells in the cat. *Quart. J. exp. Physiol.*, **1958**, *44*: 1–25.

POGGIO, G.F. and MOUNTCASTLE, V.B. The functional properties of ventro-basal thalamic neurons studied in unanesthetized monkeys. *J. Neurophysiol.*, **1963**, *26*: 775–806.

PRINCE, D.A. and WILDER, B.J. Control mechanisms in cortical epileptogenic foci. "Surround" inhibition. *Arch. Neurol. (Chic.)*, **1967**, *16*: 194–202.

PURPURA, D.P. and COHEN, B. Intracellular recording from thalamic neurons during recruiting responses. *J. Neurophysiol.*, **1962**, *25*: 621–635.

ROSENBLUETH, A. and CANNON, W.B. Cortical responses to electric stimulation. *Amer. J. Physiol.*, **1941–42**, *135*: 690–741.

SAWA, M., MARUYAMA, N. and KAJI, S. Intracellular potential during electrically induced seizures. *Electroenceph. clin. Neurophysiol.*, **1963**, *15*: 209–220.

SAWA, M., NAKAMURA, K. and NAITO, H. Intracellular phenomena and spread of epileptic seizure discharges. *Electroenceph. clin. Neurophysiol.*, **1968**, *24*: 146–154.

SUGAYA, E., GOLDRING, S. and O'LEARY, J. Intracellular potentials associated with direct cortical response and seizure discharge in cat. *Electroenceph. clin. Neurophysiol.*, **1964**, *17*: 661–669.

WILDER, B.J. and MORRELL, F. Cellular behavior in secondary epileptic lesions. *Neurology (Minneap.)*, **1967**, *17*: 1193–1204.

YAMAMOTO, S. Unit activation in temporal cortex during amygdaloid seizures in cats. *Electroenceph. clin. Neurophysiol.*, **1963**, *15*: 221–229.

YOKOTA, T. and MacLEAN, P.D. Inhibitory effect of hippocampal seizures on unit responses evoked by fifth nerve stimulation in squirrel monkeys. *Electroenceph. clin. Neurophysiol.*, **1968**, *24*: 190P.

Mechanisms of Neuronal Hyperexcitability [1]

ARTHUR A. WARD Jr.

Department of Neurological Surgery, University of Washington School of Medicine, Seattle, Washington 98105 (U.S.A.)

Although our knowledge of the general phenomenon of epilepsy is unfortunately fragmentary, our best data at the present time deal with the properties of seizures of focal onset in the cerebral cortex. Focal seizures of cortical origin have provided the most definitive data in the human, and the majority of research in experimental animals has been directed at seizures induced in the cortex by a variety of means. In these circumstances, the general phenomenon is thought to consist of an epileptogenic focus consisting of a cluster of hyperactive neurons whose individual members exhibit certain patterns of firing and which collectively generate the epileptic spike as recorded with gross electrodes. There is general agreement that the latter represents the hallmark of the epileptic process. This epileptic spike occurs at random intervals during the long inter-ictal periods while, at times, the focus generates a propagating seizure discharge which results in a clinical seizure. Both the inter-ictal as well as ictal events constitute the general phenomenon called epilepsy. However, there are reasons for believing that the mechanisms involved in the propagation of the seizure discharge may be quite different from those generating the inter-ictal activity at the focus. Thus the use of the generic term epilepsy, which includes both processess, has tended to confuse hypotheses regarding mechanism, has led to semantic ambiguities, and has even tended to entangle concepts developed from data on various experimental models. Thus studies of electrically induced after-discharge may provide useful insight into the mechanisms involved in the spread or propagation of an epileptic seizure, but may have little relevance to the mechanisms generating the inter-ictal activity at the epileptogenic focus.

In focal cortical epilepsy, the essential feature is the epileptogenic focus since, in its absence, a propagating seizure does not arise. The primary concern is then to try and determine the biological characteristics of the focus and identify the complex mechanisms generating the inter-ictal hyperactivity. Since our scientific heritage commits us to an analytical approach, we inevitably come to the goal of trying to determine the mechanisms generating the pathological hyperactivity of a single epileptic neuron. Such a strategy presumes that the epileptogenic focus is composed of an unspecified number of such prototype "epileptic neurons", the necessary critical mass being unknown at the present time although it is clearly more than one.

[1] This work was supported by Public Health Service Research Grant NB-04053 from the National Institute of Neurological Diseases and Stroke.

References pp. 85–86

THE EPILEPTIC NEURON

The behavior of single neurons in the epileptogenic focus has been examined in a variety of experimental models in which the seizure process has usually been acutely induced. Our efforts, however, have been largely directed at studies involving spontaneous seizure activity in chronic epileptogenic foci in the monkey. These foci are induced by the subpial injection of aluminum hydroxide into the sensori-motor cortex which is followed, after 4–12 weeks, by the occurrence of spontaneous clinical seizures. The clinical pattern of the seizures is characteristic of the location of the scar as in human epilepsy of focal cortical onset. The seizures occur spontaneously, and frequency is roughly proportional to the degree of cortical pathology induced. Once established, the clinical seizures recur spontaneously for many years with a relatively constant pattern of seizure frequency. Although we have confined our studies to foci induced in the monkey, it has recently been noted that similar foci can be induced in the cat (Schmalbach 1970).

In monkeys exhibiting spontaneous clinical seizures, the epileptogenic focus is characterized by the occurrence of EEG spikes as recorded from either the scalp or the exposed cortex. It is then possible to monitor the activity of single neurons in the focus by extracellular recording utilizing tungsten micro-electrodes introduced trans-

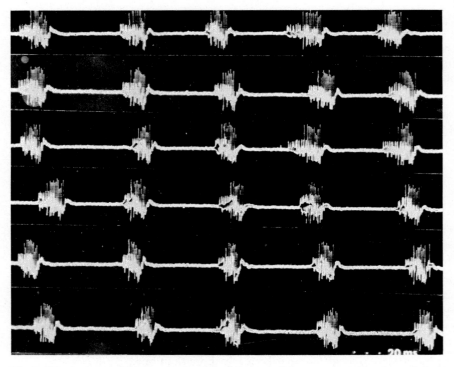

Fig. 1. Rhythmic repetitive bursts recorded with extracellular tungsten microelectrode from epileptic focus in awake, undrugged monkey. Samples of activity from same unit recorded over a period of 6 h. (From Sypert and Ward, unpublished data.)

durally through an implanted chamber in awake, undrugged monkeys. The most frequently encountered pattern of inter-ictal discharge is recurrent, high frequency bursts of action potentials (Fig. 1). Firing rates in a burst may vary from 200–900/sec; the burst starts at high frequency and there is no decrement in frequency during the burst. There are few if any spikes between bursts; the bursts repeat 5–15 times/sec. The bursts are stereotyped, showing little fluctuation in the first few spikes of the burst. An exception is a special type of burst with a structured timing pattern that has been observed only within the area of major spike activity as recorded in the surface EEG at the focus. The pattern of firing within these special bursts is characterized by a long first interval between the first and subsequent spikes in the burst. The fine structure of the timing within such bursts has been examined by Calvin *et al.* (1968) utilizing computer techniques. These long-first-interval neurons seem to have two components to their bursts: a first spike and a group of stereotyped spikes beginning with the second spike. Neither appears alone, always being infallibly associated with each other. The long first interval can be remarkably fixed in duration or it can be quite variable, in some cases with a bimodal behavior. The rest of the burst which follows is merely

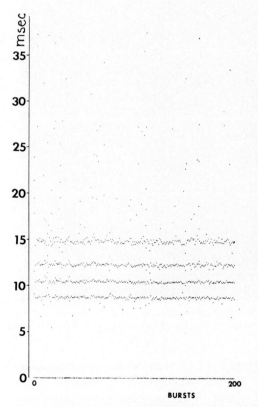

Fig. 2. Raster display of 200 consecutive spontaneous epileptic bursts recorded in awake, undrugged monkey. Each dot represents one spike in a burst; each vertical row is one burst. Successive bursts are horizontally aligned next to each other, to aid in visually judging burst patterns. (From Calvin, Sypert and Ward, unpublished data.)

stereotyped and locked to the second spike. Fig. 2 represents a computer generated raster display of the patterns of firing in the bursts of such an epileptic neuron. Here each dot represents a spike and the first spikes of each of the bursts are lined up at the bottom. Subsequent spikes in a burst are plotted immediately above each other. This permits a large amount of raw data to be compacted so that it can be scanned visually to check for patterns of firing within the bursts. It is seen that there is an interval of 8.6 msec between the first and subsequent spikes which repeat at approximately 1.6 msec intervals. The long first interval is remarkably constant.

Thus the behavior of epileptic neurons is characterized by spontaneous rhythmic burst firing. The bursts are composed of high frequency firing for 10–40 msec with few if any spikes between the bursts. The bursts repeat 7–15 times/sec. The bursts tend to be stereotyped except for some which have special properties of timing characterized by a long first interval.

Patterns of firing of single neuronal elements in the epileptogenic focus of man have also been examined during the course of operations for epilepsy (Ward 1969). Patterns of high frequency firing in bursts have been recorded (Fig. 3) which are indistinguish-

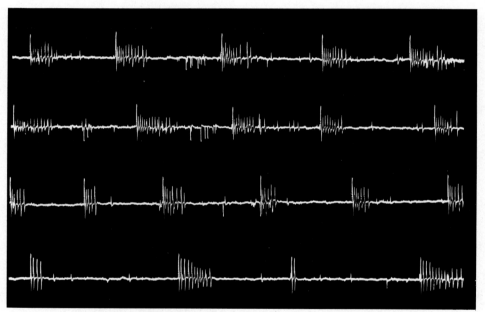

Fig. 3. Rhythmic repetitive bursts of epileptic neuron recorded in epileptic focus of human temporal lobe. Samples of activity from same cell over a period of 15 min. (From Ward and Ojemann, unpublished data.)

able from those recorded in the awake, undrugged monkey. In the more limited human data, the bursts tend to be less stereotyped than those recorded in the monkey model and, as yet, no long-first-interval bursts have been observed in the human. However, such computer analysis requires long periods of stable recording which are much more difficult to achieve in the human because of technical limitations imposed by the clinical setting.

Such patterns of burst firing do not appear to be characteristic of the behavior of normal cortical neurons and may have synaptic consequences not ordinarily considered in our models of the transmission of signals in the central nervous system. The current model of neuronal firing states that steady-state net depolarizations are converted into the firing rate of that neuron and then back into net depolarizations at the next synapse. This "amplitude-to-frequency" model is supported by many studies of repetitive firing of cat spinal motoneurons and of cat cortical neurons. Under these circumstances, unless the depolarization exceeds a minimum level, few spikes occur. When rhythmic firing does begin, it jumps from zero to an elevated rate called the "minimum rhythmic firing rate". The firing rate then increases in direct proportion to further increments in the depolarizing currents from the synapses. A general theory of post-synaptic potential (PSP) summation has recently been developed by Calvin (1971) and he has applied this to bursting synaptic inputs such as those generated by epileptic neurons (Calvin 1972).

Calvin has utilized an analog cable model and LINC–8 digital computer to simulate the phenomenon. It is well known that a train of spikes in a pre-synaptic pathway generates PSPs in the post-synaptic neuron which will begin to sum. However, this sum does not keep building up indefinitely because the membrane potential depolarization will decay at a rate proportional to the elevation above the baseline. Thus with repetitive firing in the pre-synaptic pathway, the final steady-state membrane potential of the post-synaptic neuron is reached as rapidly as a single PSP decays. As Calvin (1971) points out, its amplitude above the baseline is a product of PSP area and mean PSP rate. Non-rhythmic patterns of spike firing contribute to greater fluctuations about this mean depolarization in the post-synaptic neuron, but do not change the envelope shape or the final steady-state average depolarization attained.

The depolarization induced by a single synapse can be estimated from available data. Single fiber PSPs have been studied in cat spinal motoneuron where they attain a height of 0.5 mV (or less) and may decay exponentially with a 5 msec time constant. A typical active input can produce 20 spikes/sec. Thus, in Calvin's model (1971), the mean depolarization would be only 50 µV, 10% of the peak height. However, given 200 such synapses, a net average depolarization of 10 mV could be attained which is about the threshold for firing the post-synaptic cell. Thus 2% of a motoneuron's 10,000 synapses firing asynchronously could either elicit rhythmic firing from a silent cell, or markedly increase a pre-existing firing rate. Since group Ia afferents account for only 2% of the synaptic inputs on a spinal motoneuron, the fact that the knee jerk can be elicited with ease indicates that this small number of synapses can be most effective. Furthermore, the data indicate that roughly 4 times this steady depolarization can often drive a cell to its high frequency firing range. Thus 8% of a motoneuron's inputs, firing at a nominal 20/sec each, could drive the cell to high firing rates. Since a neuron in the motor cortex of the monkey has 60,000 synapses, presumably 1.3% of its synapses firing at nominal rates could generate high frequency firing.

Epileptic neurons, on the other hand, instead of firing at 20/sec often fire at rates of 200–900/sec during their bursts which may last from 10–40 msec or longer. Assuming 200/sec rates within an epileptic burst, the previous example now requires only

20 synapses with overlapping bursts to be capable of significantly disrupting the normal activities of the post-synaptic neuron. Thus, by Calvin's computation, a mere 80 bursting input boutons would be sufficient to cause high frequency firing in the post-synaptic cell. Thus only 0.13% of the 60,000 synapses of a cortical neuron need to be bursting to convert this cell into another bursting cell.

If one applies the computation of PSP summation to the timing patterns of actual epileptic bursts, Calvin has indicated the PSP burst summation for 3 different PSP shapes, corresponding to synaptic locations at 0.0, 0.5 and 1.0 space constants from the recording site as indicated in Fig. 4. It is apparent that the epileptic burst is a very efficient "packaging" compared to the firing patterns of normal cortical neurons. This is further indicated in Fig. 5 where the computer predicts the PSPs generated by a normal cortical neuron firing at 40–60/sec and compares this with the predicted PSP summation generated by an epileptic neuron firing at approximately the same average rate. It is apparent that concentrating the spikes into bursts produces higher depolarizations. Thus, with perhaps 40–100 bursting inputs, a bursting response is predicted in the post-synaptic cell. Such secondary bursts will be somewhat delayed, due to the time required for the PSP envelope to rise through the threshold region. The longer

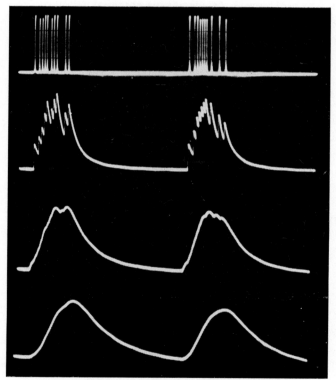

Fig. 4. PSP summation predicted for epileptic burst spike patterns. *Top trace:* burst firing of epileptic neuron in monkey. *Second trace:* predicted temporal summation from a "nearby" synapse with a decay time constant of 10 msec. *Third* and *lowest traces:* predicted temporal summation at time constants of 0.5 and 1.0 sec respectively, normalized in amplitude to match second trace (decay time constants 35 and 60 msec) (Calvin 1971).

the input bursts, the greater the possibility of the responding bursts overlapping in time with them, and thus the greater the potential of the recruited neuron for contributing to further burst recruitment of still other normal cells.

A group of such primary epileptic bursting neurons in the center of an epileptic focus might be expected to have an appreciable density of synaptic connections to normal neurons in the surrounding cortex allowing recruitment of normal neurons to widen the extent of the "focus". Background synaptic activity should bias such recruitment. Thus bursting inputs which are subliminal to some normal neurons will begin to cause firing when the background depolarization from synaptic input from other sources takes care of the first 10 mV of membrane depolarization. On this basis, the size of the epileptic focus should expand and shrink depending upon background synaptic activity and upon synchronizing factors.

These problems of recruitment make it somewhat difficult to experimentally distinguish between the "primary" or pacemaker epileptic neurons and the "follower" normal neurons which receive this optimal bursting input in less than 0.5% of the synapses ending upon them. The data obtained by Prince and Futamachi (1968) from intracellular recording in the chronic epileptic focus of the monkey showed burst firing occuring at the peak of large membrane depolarizations which are very similar to the summed PSPs in follower neurons (Fig. 5) predicted by Calvin's computer simulation (1971). Even with extracellular recording, these summed PSPs may be reflected by field potentials which can be occasionally observed to be temporally related to the burst firing (Ward 1969). With these concepts in mind, additional data in the future may provide a basis for establishing clearer criteria to distinguish the firing patterns of primary epileptic neurons from the bursts generated in follower normal neurons.

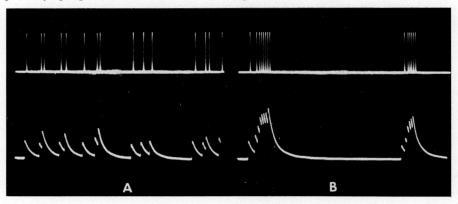

Fig. 5. Predicted temporal summation for normal and epileptic spike patterns. *A:* normal cortical neuron firing at relatively high, irregular rate and its predicted PSP in postsynaptic cell. *B:* epileptic neuron firing at approximately the same average rate but in bursts. It is apparent that concentrating the spikes into bursts produces higher depolarizations in the postsynaptic cell (Calvin 1971).

Morphologically, the chronic epileptogenic focus in both monkey and man is characterized by depopulation of neurons and the remaining neurons appear to be of small size. There is a striking astrocytic gliosis in which the epileptic neurons are embedded. The epileptic neurons are characterized, in Golgi stained sections, by a striking loss of dendritic spines and other changes in dendritic structure (Westrum *et al.* 1965). Similar studies of neurons in human foci also indicate that loss of dendritic spines is a characteristic attribute of epileptic neurons (Scheibel and Scheibel 1968). These modifications of morphological structures dealing with input to the neuron are of interest since it has been repeatedly observed that it is most difficult to evoke the characteristic high frequency burst activity of epileptic neurons in sensory cortex by sensory volleys. Thus one might propose that epileptic neurons are partially denervated. It is unlikely that all synaptic input is lost since epileptic seizures in the human and monkey can be modified by events that are, presumably, synaptically mediated. However, such effects might be mediated by synaptic input on the nearby follower neurons that are intermittently recruited into burst activity.

The thesis that a reduction in synaptic input can result in autonomous hyperactivity is difficult to test directly in the cerebral cortex where it is not possible to divorce afferent from efferent activity because of the complex geometry of the cortical feltwork. However, we have examined this problem at lower levels in the central nervous system. The spinal trigeminal system lends itself well to a study of neuronal deafferentation since it is supplied by a large nerve containing only sensory fibers. If one monitors the spontaneous activity of the first order neuron in the spinal trigeminal complex in the brain stem at varying periods of time after retro-Gasserian rhizotomy, dramatic hyperactivity can be recorded (Ward 1969). This hyperactivity first appears some 10–20 days after rhizotomy and by 19 days neurons are observed to be firing in brief bursts separated by equally short periods of inactivity. At 31 days after rhizotomy, the hyperactivity is even more pronounced and almost uninterrupted tonic firing is encountered in neurons throughout the pars interpolaris and caudalis of the spinal trigeminal complex of the cat.

Selective alterations of afferent input can also be studied in the spinal cord. If one records the activity of single neurons in the cord 2–25 weeks after intradural rhizotomy from L5 through S1, spontaneous bursts of high frequency firing are recorded. The spontaneous hyperactivity and burst firing is most prominent in smaller neurons of the dorsal horn in laminae V, VI, and VII. Somewhat similar high frequency firing in neurons in the lumbar cord can also be induced by hemicordotomy at more cephalic levels (Loeser and Ward 1967). Limited confirmation of these data has also been obtained in man (Loeser *et al.* 1968) where the spontaneous activity of spinal neurons was sampled at the upper border of the segmental level of clinical paraplegia. Again tonic, high frequency firing was recorded.

Thus partial deafferentation of neurons in the spinal cord of animal and man or deafferentation of brain-stem neurons after trigeminal rhizotomy results in spontaneous hyperactivity. The patterns of firing of such partially deafferented neurons are qualitatively similar to the firing patterns of neurons in the epileptic focus in the cortex where there is also both physiological and anatomical evidence to indicate that the synaptic input is altered.

Unfortunately we have no direct data dealing with the structural or functional properties of denervated post-synaptic membrane in neurons of the central nervous system. We can only speculate, utilizing the models generated by the studies on denervated postjunctional membrane in muscle. It appears that the membrane potential of denervated muscle falls from the neighborhood of 100 mV to 77 mV at 50 days after denervation (Ware *et al.* 1954). The alteration of functional properties of excitable cells is not a consequence of homogenous changes in the cell membrane. Rather it is a consequence of changes in the properties of localized post-synaptic patches in the membrane. Belmar and Eyzaguirre (1966) have shown that the fibrillatory potentials in denervated muscle originate from the denervated end-plate zone and that this region represents the only areas from which the generation of rhythmic discharges can be influenced. They propose that fibrillation is produced by a steady generator potential at the denervated subsynaptic sites and present data to indicate that such sites are both chemically and electrically excitable. As they point out: "It is interesting to note that in terms of fibrillary activity the membrane at the denervated end-plate zone seems to have properties different from the rest of the muscle fiber membrane. Thus cathodal currents and drugs (such as ACh and noradrenaline) increase the frequency of fibrillation only when applied to the denervated end-plate zone in spite of the fact that currents and ACh induce membrane potential changes wherever they are applied. Therefore, changes in fibrillation frequency cannot be ascribed only to membrane potential changes. The pacemaker site must have some special properties which make it different from the rest of the muscle membrane."

Thus, to recapitulate, the epileptic process ultimately is a consequence of the interictal neuronal hyperactivity of primary pacemaker neurons. Any model of the mechanisms inducing such pacemaker activity should account for certain observations. It appears that epilepsy of focal onset in the cerebral cortex is induced by damage to neurons in both the human and in the monkey models. Some weeks, months or years after such an insult, an epileptogenic focus appears and clinical seizures are observed. The focus is characterized morphologically by depopulation of neurons, and the remaining neurons appear to be of small size. There is a dense astrocytic gliosis in which the epileptic neurons are embedded; the epileptic neurons are characterized, in the Golgi stain, by a striking loss of dendritic spines and other changes in dendritic structure. Electrophysiologically, the focus is defined by the presence of "epileptic spikes" in the electrocorticogram. The activity of individual neurons in the focus typically consists of autonomous high frequency firing, often in bursts some of which have special properties of timing. There is both morphological and electrophysiological data to indicate that such epileptic neurons are partially deafferented.

It is proposed that such pacemaker or primary epileptic neurons generate repetitive firing with abnormal sites of spike generation. On the one hand, the spike generation may be confined to initial segment or, more probably to proximal axon, driven by the generator potentials of the denervated subsynaptic sites and, possibly, by mechanical deformation of the dendritic tree. On the other hand, the dendritic generator potentials might induce spikes in the dendrites. Currents of sequential spike discharges in dendrites would summate, resulting in rapid building up of a large depolarization in soma as has been described in Purkinje neurons by Fujita (1968). This large soma depolarization (known as the inactivation response in Purkinje cells) would lead to repetitive firing in the axon. In addition, the pathways for potassium efflux may be re-

References pp. 85–86

duced around the epileptic neurons as a consequence of the astrocytic gliosis. Under these circumstances, appreciable levels of local potassium accumulation would occur as Fertziger and Ranck point out (1970). If the interstitial potassium concentration exceeds a certain threshold, it may trigger a regenerative all-or-none process (Fertziger and Ranck 1970; Pollen and Trachtenberg 1970; Trachtenberg and Pollen 1970). These mechanisms have been presented in some detail by Pollen earlier in this symposium. Thus, given the presence of generator potentials, the induction of high frequency burst firing could easily be a consequence of these several processes. The high frequency firing during the burst is followed by a relatively long period of electrical silence before the next burst. This suppression of repetitive firing could be accounted for by a variety of mechanisms including post-tetanic hyperpolarization due to activation of an electrogenic sodium pump in the soma (Nakajima and Takahashi 1966) or by recurrent collateral inhibition. Both of these mechanisms could effectively time the bursts. Thus this model proposes that orthodromic burst firing in pacemaker epileptic neurons is induced by generator potentials in dendrites and other mechanisms operating upon abnormal sites of spike generation.

In addition, antidromic firing may be induced in either the same or other epileptic neurons of the focus by a site of spike generation in the terminal axons. It is known that, subsequent to conditioning by a high frequency volley, axons respond to a single spike with brief trains of repetitive action potentials. It is thought that the tetanic conditioning volley induces hyperpolarization of the terminal branches of the axon (Rang and Ritchie 1968). Under such circumstances, the arrival of a single spike induces a repetitive discharge which is antidromically conducted back up the axon. This post-tetanic hyperpolarization appears to be a consequence of activation of an electrogenic sodium pump (Rang and Ritchie 1968). This mechanism accounts not only for post-tetanic repetitive firing in axons but is also invoked as the mechanism for the post-tetanic potentiation (PTP) of muscle response and the PTP of the monosynaptic reflex in the spinal cord. Furthermore, post-tetanic hyperpolarization is augmented by increases in extracellular potassium and such increases in K efflux have been demonstrated in the epileptic focus by Fertziger and Ranck (1970) during experimentally induced seizures. It is of interest that one of the best documented physiological actions of the well known anti-convulsant drug diphenylhydantoin is to suppress both post-tetanic repetitive firing (Raines and Standaert 1966) and PTP in the cord (Esplin 1957).

If mechanisms in the epileptic focus could induce hyperpolarization of the presynaptic terminals by activation of an electrogenic Na pump, then a single spike originating in a somewhat distant normal neuron would evoke a repetitive discharge in these terminals as in the case of post-tetanic repetitive firing. If the monitoring extracellular electrode is located close to the distant cell body, one would record the initial spike and the returning antidromic burst generated in the preterminal fibers. The first spike would be separated from the burst by an interval determined by the round-trip conduction velocity and could account for the long-first-interval burst recorded in epileptic neurons (Calvin *et al.* 1968).

Other mechanisms could equally well evoke such antidromic activity in axon terminals. Presynaptic inhibition is thought to operate *via* synapses upon the presynaptic terminals of an axon. These synapses depolarize the terminals which is thought to reduce the average quantity of transmitter released when a spike arrives. However, such presynaptic depolarization, if strong enough to cross threshold, could itself initiate a spike which would then propagate antidromically up the axon. This is considered to be the basis for the dorsal root reflex (Wall 1964). If one further assumes that the neurons providing such presynaptic inhibitory input are small, internuncial pacemaker cells in the focus, a potent source of presynaptic depolarization might be generated to evoke such firing in axon terminals of a more distant, relatively healthy neuron.

In addition, a site of spike generation in the terminal axons of the pacemaker epileptic neurons themselves could generate such bursts. Recent reports have indicated that antidromic stimulation of cat spinal motoneurons induces, when properly conditioned, a centrifugal discharge in Group I primary afferent fibers (Decima and Goldberg 1969). This phenomenon of neuron-presynaptic coupling might be grossly augmented in the epileptic focus. Under such circumstances, the spontaneous firing of the follower cell could induce a spike in the axon terminals of the presynaptic pacemaker neuron. This antidromically conducted spike would now evoke a burst of repetitive firing in the pacemaker cell. If the site of the recording electrode is close to the post-synaptic follower cell, it would record the initial, normal spike (evoking the antidromic impulse) followed, after an interval determined by round-trip conduction velocity and synaptic delay, by a repetitive burst. Thus the bursts would be characterized by a long first interval. At other times, the burst firing might be generated in the pacemaker neuron by mechanisms proposed above and orthodromically conducted down the axon driving the follower neuron into burst activity. The recorded burst would then be a nonspecific burst without such special properties of intra-burst timing such as the long first interval. Our data are still limited, but it appears that both classes of neurons can be observed in the focus. As previously reported (Calvin *et al.* 1968), long-first-interval bursts can be the only behavior recorded in some cells. More recently, it appears that some cells may alternate between long-first-interval behavior and non-specific burst behavior. This model would provide mechanisms for both types of behavior.

The details of synaptic organization from a morphological as well as a physiological standpoint are currently poorly understood in normal cortex. It is then inevitable that we can only speculate regarding the mechanisms generating neuronal hyperactivity in a pathological state known as epilepsy. However, the current meager data are now making it possible to construct some fairly definitive models which can be subjected to experimental test. In the course of such an endeavor, not only will the models undergo appreciable refinement but it is possible that such studies will also throw new light on normal synaptic mechanisms in the cerebral cortex.

REFERENCES

BELMAR, J. and EYZAGUIRRE, C. Pacemaker site of fibrillation potentials in denervated mammalian muscle. *J. Neurophysiol.*, **1966**, *29*: 425–441.

CALVIN, W. H. Synaptic potential summation and repetitive firing mechanisms: input–output theory for the recruitment of neurons into epileptic bursting firing patterns. *Brain Res.*, **1972** (in press).

CALVIN, W.H., SYPERT, G.W. and WARD JR., A.A. Structured timing patterns within bursts from epileptic neurons in undrugged monkey cortex. *Exp. Neurol.*, **1968**, *21*: 535–549.

DECIMA, E. E. and GOLDBERG, L. J. Time course of excitability changes of primary afferent terminals as determined by monosynaptic-presynaptic interaction. *Brain Res.*, **1969**, *15*: 288–290.

ESPLIN, D.W. Effects of diphenylhydantoin on synaptic transmission in cat spinal cord and stellate ganglion. *J. Pharmacol. exp. Ther.*, **1957**, *120*: 301–323.

FERTZIGER, A.P. and RANCK JR., J.B. Potassium accumulation in interstitial space during epileptiform seizures. *Exp. Neurol.*, **1970**, *26*: 571–585.

FUJITA, Y. Activity of dendrites of single Purkinje cells and its relationship to so-called inactivation response in rabbit cerebellum. *J. Neurophysiol.*, **1968**, *31*: 131–141.

LOESER, J.D. and WARD JR., A.A. Some effects of deafferentation on neurons of the cat spinal cord. *Arch. Neurol., (Chic.)*, **1967**, *17*: 629–636.

LOESER, J.D., WARD JR., A.A. and WHITE, L.E. Chronic deafferentation of human spinal cord neurons. *J. Neurosurg.*, **1968**, *29*: 48–50.

NAKAJIMA, S. and TAKAHASHI, K. Post-tetanic hyperpolarization and electrogenic pump in stretch receptor neurone of crayfish. *J. Physiol. (Lond.)*, **1966**, *187*: 105–127.

POLLEN, D.A. and TRACHTENBERG, M.C. Neuroglia: gliosis and focal epilepsy. *Science*, **1970**, *167*: 1252–1253.

PRINCE, D.A. and FUTAMACHI, K.J. Intracellular recordings in chronic focal epilepsy. *Brain Res.*, **1968**, *11*: 681–684.

RAINES, A. and STANDAERT, F.G. Pre- and postjunctional effects of diphenylhydantoin at the cat soleus neuromuscular junction. *J. Pharmacol. exp. Ther.*, **1966**, *153*: 361-366.

RANG, H.P. and RITCHIE, J.M. On the electrogenic sodium pump in mammalian non-myelinated nerve fibers and its activation by various external cations. *J. Physiol. (Lond.)*, **1968**, *196*: 183–221.

SCHEIBEL, M.E. and SCHEIBEL, A.B. On the nature of dendritic spines: report of a workshop. *Communic. Behav. Biol.*, **1968**, *1*: 231.

SCHMALBACH, K. An animal model of the epileptic process. *Pharmakopsych. Neuro-pharm.*, **1970**, *3*: 161–175.

TRACHTENBERG, M.C. and POLLEN, D.A. Neuroglia: biophysical properties and physiological function. *Science*, **1970**, *167*: 1248–1252.

WALL, P.D. Presynaptic control of impulses at the first central synapse in the cutaneous pathway. In J.C. ECCLES and J.P. SCHADÉ (EDS.), *Progress in brain research, Vol. 12. Physiology of spinal neurons*. Elsevier, Amsterdam, **1964**: 92–115.

WARD JR., A.A. The epileptic neuron: chronic foci in animals and man. In H.H. JASPER, A.A. WARD JR. and A. POPE (EDS.), *Basic mechanisms of the epilepsies*. Little, Brown, Boston, **1969**: 263–288.

WARE JR. F., BENNETT, A.L. and McINTYRE, A.R. Membrane resting potential of denervated mammalian skeletal muscle measured *in vivo. Amer. J. Physiol.*, **1954**, *177*: 115–118.

WESTRUM, L.E., WHITE JR., L.E. and WARD JR. A.A. Morphology of the experimental epileptic focus. *J. Neurosurg.*, **1965**, *21*: 1033–1046.

Akinesia paradoxica[1]

ROBERT S. SCHWAB

Massachusetts General Hospital, Boston, Mass. 02114 (U.S.A.)

Of all the very puzzling clinical phenomena met with in Parkinson's disease, akinesia paradoxica is the most unusual and difficult to explain on any rational anatomical basis.

Before describing akinesia paradoxica (perhaps better termed kinesia paradoxica) we should define the term akinesia which is very common and surely the most disabling of all Parkinsonian symptoms. Physicians are very familiar with the typical resting 5/-sec tremor of this disorder and to the resistance of the muscles to passive manipulation covered by the term rigidity. Indeed some have called Parkinson's disease a tremor-rigidity syndrome. Most of the therapeutic efforts in the past, going back to Charcot's orginal use of belladonna alkaloids 100 years ago through the synthetic modern compounds and the various attempts of basal ganglia surgical intervention, have been strongly focussed on the abolition or reduction of the tremor and the rigidity. There has been little success and inadequate attention paid to this far more disabling symptom called akinesia, which can be characterized as follows:

(*1*) Akinesia is a severe difficulty on the part of the patient in initiating a voluntary motor activity. There is not only a delay in starting, but if it is to continue at all it must occupy the entire attention of the person. The poverty of movement typical of the disease is due partly to this akinesia associated with the difficulty in initiating motor patterns.

(*2*) There is a difficulty in altering movements smoothly and efficiently which we ordinarily expect in a normal. For example, a walking Parkinsonian patient who has to turn at a right angle very often stumbles or delays his turn and has difficulty in making it.

(*3*) There is difficulty in stopping the motor activity at a precise moment when it would be most efficient and desirable. Overshooting and running into objects in walking are examples.

(*4*) The most difficult of all is maintaining a normal or desired amplitude of the motor activity involved. This is the most disabling and disastrous to the patient of any of the features of the akinesia. The patient may start out with a normal 18 in. stride in walking, but very rapidly the distance is reduced until the feet cover no more than a few inches at each stride, upsetting the normal balance and producing various tendencies to fall and propel the patient into a run. The handwriting will rapidly diminish in size until it becomes micrographic and illegible (Fig. 1).

[1] Supported in part by a grant from the Allen P. and Josephine B. Green Foundation, Mexico, Missouri, U.S.A.

References p. 92

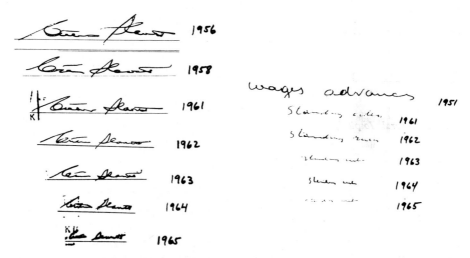

Fig. 1. Samples of signature of 2 patients with Parkinson's disease. Date of onset of disease in patient on left was 1959. Handwriting already showed reduced size 1 year before. In 1965 there was bilateral akinesia with more rigidity on the dominant right side. Patient on right began his disease in 1960. Writing in 1965 was illegible, and speech inaudible. There was marked akinesia and moderate bilateral rigidity.

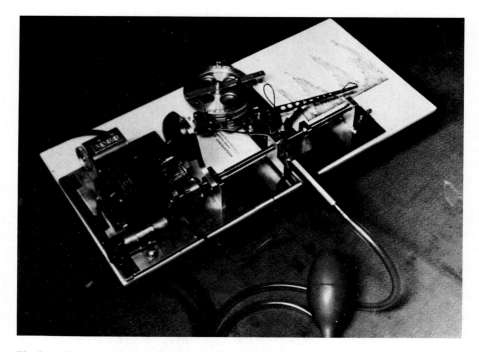

Fig. 2. Bulb ergograph made by Mr. Fred Christensen, 11 Wilmot St., Watertown, Mass., U.S.A. At 1 revolution/sec, pen carriage moves 1 mm. Bell rings each second. On this model there is an integrator (EcK work adder) of total pen excursion as well as a revolution counter.

Speech is audible for the first few syllables, but the amplitude falls off and soon leaves the speaker's voice inaudible and, of course, not understandable.

We have been very much interested in the akinesia occurring in this disease for the past 20 years in particular. Since 1949 we have been using a simple bulb ergograph (Fig. 2) in the regular testing of all Parkinsonian patients to study the phenomenon of akinesia with some objective measurements. A normal person can squeeze this bulb actuating the ergographic pen at 1/sec intervals for 1 min without a loss of amplitude, and we have many hundreds of normal tracings of the sort seen in Fig. 3. Even if the

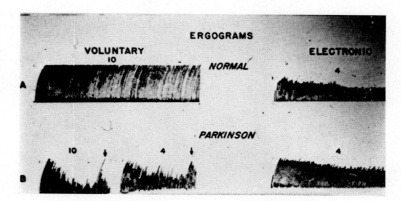

Fig. 3. Examples of ergograms. *A*: normal subject. On the left: voluntary movement, moving a 10 g weight (modification of ergograph; right adductor pollicis muscle). Right: same muscle driven electrically with high voltage Batrow glass stimulator with 4 g weight. Note inferior performance with electronic ergograph in normal person. *B*: Parkinsonian patient. On the left: 2 voluntary ergograms with 10 and 4 g weights; the arrow shows supreme effort. Right: electronic ergogram of the same patient and same muscle, 4 g weight. Electronic ergogram is normal and much better than with voluntary effort.

person complains of muscular fatigue towards the end of this minute he can maintain full amplitude whether he watches the pen or whether he just continues to squeeze the bulb. Longer periods of more than 1 min at full amplitude will result in a gradual decline of amplitude in a normal fatigue process.

The Parkinsonian patient produces in the early evolution of the disorder slight amounts of amplitude fatigue that are more extreme than normal. As the disease progresses, however, the drop off in the amplitude then becomes a conspicuous characteristic of the disease. The presence of rigidity in the muscles of the arm being tested accentuates this early fatigue and produces akinesia directly related to the rigidity. The presence of tremor has little effect on the ergograph until it is severe enough to mechanically interfere with proper squeezing of the bulb. When the disease becomes bilateral the degree of this amplitude reduction becomes progressively greater until advanced cases present curves that reach the zero line within fractions of a minute. Indeed their initial excursion is also much less than the normal.

These typical and marked fatigue ergograms suggest that the Parkinson muscle is in various states of exhaustion such as seen in motor neuritis, myasthenia gravis, etc. Electro-ergograms were used by us in 1952 and we were able to show then that a

References p. 92

Parkinsonian patient with marked muscular amplitude reduction could have the same muscle driven electrically without any evidence of fatigue (Fig. 3).

With this fact in mind we began to develop various techniques in raising the stimulus directed at the patient so that motivation would be increased and better performance result. We have already shown that the degree of handicap and the effects of stress varied according to the personality type of the patient rather than to the degree of rigidity and tremor (Prichard and Schwab 1951). When fatigue appears in the ergograph in a Parkinsonian patient, the nurse can shout at the patient to increase his amplitude and he usually will do so (Fig. 4). The fatigue, however, immediately recurs.

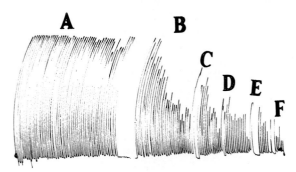

Fig. 4. Bulb ergograms 1/sec. *A*: normal control, right hand. *B–F*: Parkinsonian, right hand. At *C* supreme effort for silver pill box prize. *D*: a second prize is offered. At *E* prize is doubled. At *F* the patient urged to duplicate *D* for gold box. He barely achieved this.

The next stimulus will not be as effective and must be increased by presenting the patient with a prize. Again it falls off and the prize has to be doubled, and so on until the end of the minute is achieved. This is shown in the parts of the ergograms *B*, *C*, *D*, *E* and *F* in Fig. 4 (Schwab and Zieper 1965).

Since this stimulus intensity effect is proportional to the improvement in the ergogram it can be measured, and percentages of the akinesia estimated. It is also apparent that there is a close resemblance to these mild degrees of improvement in motor performance by increasing motivation to the phenomenon which we will now describe as akinesia paradoxica or as it was called by Bing (1923) kinesia paradoxica. This phenomenon was extensively studied and measured by Kinnier Wilson who described it in his Croonian Lectures in 1925, and it has been amply documented in various reports since that time. It is defined as a sudden total loss of akinesia lasting somewhere under one minute in time that occurs as a result of a catastrophe. A few examples will illustrate the point.

Case 1. A 61-year-old woman with advanced bilateral, totally disabling Parkinson's disease had become restricted to a wheel chair existence, requiring full time attendance of her daughter and nurse in the home where a 1-year-old grand-daughter resided. The patient lived on the second floor of the house. One night while the infant's parents were away briefly the house caught fire, burning briskly with great columns of smoke. The patient jumped out of her wheel chair, grabbed the baby in her arms and ran down the stairs to the arriving firemen, and then collapsed back to her state of total invalidism. While no one witnessed the initial motor patterns of this extraordinary phenomenon, the terminal part was amply documented. Only estimates can be made of the total duration of this apparent return of full motor ability for this brief period of time.

Case 2. A 58-year-old male with advanced bilateral Parkinson's disease for the previous 3 years had been a total invalid, unable to go upstairs, dress or feed himself. His wife arranged for him to live on the first floor of their home in Providence. In the middle of September 1960, in a howling rainstorm, she left him to go shopping. One of the Caribbean hurricanes, Donna, came up the coast and piled up a 12-foot tide. This wall of water crashed into the door of this patient's home. Three hours later the police who arrived by boat found him on the second floor, collapsed in a chair, unable to move and, according to his wife, his feet were not even wet. This miraculous return of his ability to run rapidly upstairs was not witnessed by anybody, but an average estimate would surely place the time as under 1 minute.

Case. 3. This has been documented by a motion picture film and occurred years ago in the Bellevue Hospital, New York, where a well known baseball pitcher was totally disabled by Parkinson's disease. His neurologist wanted to demonstrate the fact that such a helpless invalid in a wheel chair could probably raise his arms and catch a ball thrown to him in an act called akinesia paradoxica. This was done with the motion picture film; surprisingly enough the patient not only caught the ball, but got out of his wheel chair and threw it back to the doctor, knocking him to the floor.

There are strange undercurrents of tradition, belief and gossip concerning nursing-home disasters in Great Britain, the United States and Australia. This involves the fact that in nursing homes which have disastrous fires the Parkinsonian patients invariably get out of the burning buildings as opposed to patients with strokes, and other total invalids. Various degrees of partial akinesia paradoxica occur from time to time in the severely handicapped patients. A sudden ringing of the telephone during the early morning hours may bring the Parkinsonian patient bounding out of bed to answer the phone, a feat he has not done for some years. One of my patients in the hospital using a bedpan in his room was suddenly confronted by three female visitors who were looking for another patient. He was able to scream at them to get out and close the door and this was loud enough to be heard at the nurse's desk. These were the first sounds he had uttered that were audible for over a year.

Parkinsonian patients frequently have great difficulty in swallowing their food without choking and in coughing efficiently as symptoms of the akinesia syndrome. I have encountered numerous times such patients who develop a threat to their trachea by a bolus of food, naturally panic and immediately expel it by a vigorous efficient cough. I have gone so far as to reassure over-anxious spouses that it is exceedingly unlikely that the patient would choke to death over an ordinary aspirated piece of food because of the saving characteristic of akinesia paradoxica in such catastrophic emergencies.

Since the accepted anatomical degeneration in this disease is in the substantia nigra where the cells lose their pigment, become atrophied and shrink, one is at a great loss to explain this dramatic sudden disappearance of the disability under catastrophic stimulation. One can only infer that there must be multiple pathways for the execution

References p. 92

of learned motor patterns such as walking, running, talking, riding, using the hands in the performance of various motor tasks, etc. In Parkinson's disease, therefore, one has to assume, if there are two alternative pathways and one is interfered with through "blocking by defective neuro-transmitters or other biochemical means" that the other, unused except in emergencies, is open and ready to go if the stimulus is sufficiently high. Where these alternative pathways are and through what basal ganglia and nuclei the impulses flow is surely not known today.

Since this symposium honoring Dr. Herbert Jasper is largely oriented to the neurophysiological sphere, this clinical report was put together for the main purpose of bringing these facts to the attention of all of our important neurophysiological colleagues here assembled and of offering them a real challenge to experiment, test and devise reasonable biochemical, physiological and pathological explanations for this extraordinary phenomenon encountered by my neurological colleagues who follow many of these Parkinsonian patients.

The brief abolition of akinesia may, as was suggested after the meeting by R. Broughton, be mediated by an inhibitory descending pathway which briefly releases normal motor patterns from the chains of the Parkinsonian invalid state (Tassinari et al. 1965). In any case, a real breakthrough even more substantial than that associated with L-dopa treatment might follow a better understanding of this remarkable phenomenon.

Note added in proof.
The term *Kinesia Paradoxica* as reported by Bing is more exact than *Akinesia Paradoxica*. There also are neurologists at present who use *Akinesia Paradoxica* to mean a sudden temporary *increase in Akinesia* during therapy with L-dopa.

REFERENCES

BING, R. Über einige bemerkenswerte Begleiterscheinungen der "extra-pyramidalen Rigidität" (Akathisie-Mikrographie-Kinesia paradoxica). *Schweiz. med. Wschr.*, **1923**, 7: 167.
KINNIER WILSON, S.A. The Croonian Lectures on some disorders of motility and of muscle tone with special reference to the corpus striatum. *Lancet*, **1925**, pp. 1, 53, 169, 215.
PRICHARD, J.S. and SCHWAB, R.S. Effects of stress and results of medication in different personalities with Parkinson's disease. *Psychosom. Med.*, **1951**, *13*: 106.
SCHWAB, R.S. and ZIEPER, I. Effects of mood, motivation, stress and alertness on the performance in Parkinson's disease. *Psychiat. et Neurol. (Basel)*, **1965**, *150*: 345.
TASSINARI, C., BROUGHTON, R., POIRÉ, R., ROGER, J. and GASTAUT, H. *Le sommeil de nuit normal et pathologique*. Masson, Paris, **1965**.

Physiological and Clinical Studies of Microreflexes[1]

The history of electrophysiology contains many illustrations of a close analogy between electrical discharges that occur in the muscle fiber and those that can be recorded from neuronal tissue. Even with modern recording techniques, the electroencephalographer may have considerable difficulty in distinguishing pathologic discharges from the brain, such as spikes, from those that may be produced by overlying muscle. The discovery of "microreflexes", consisting of myogenic responses to afferent stimuli which are often indistinguishable from evoked cortical potentials, has further emphasized the close relation between muscle and brain. Thus, it is appropriate to dedicate this paper to Doctor Jasper who contributed importantly to both fields and early recognized the significant inter-relationships of electrical discharge in these systems.

The discovery of the evoked muscle response and its elaboration into a concept of the microreflex was made some seven years ago (Bickford 1963, 1964a; Bickford *et al.* 1964b) and work in our own and other laboratories has now indicated the important role that these phenomena may play in the elucidation of physiological mechanisms and particularly in providing significant tests of neurological function in health and disease (Bickford 1963, 1964a, b, 1966a, b, 1967; Bickford *et al.* 1963a, b, c, 1964a, b; Kiang *et al.* 1963; Cody *et al.* 1964, 1965; Jacobson *et al.* 1964a, b; Cody and Bickford 1965; Cracco and Bickford 1966a, b; Broughton *et al.* 1967; Bickford and Klass 1969; Townsend and Cody 1971).

DEFINITIONS

A microreflex may be defined as a reflex response to an afferent stimulus that requires some degree of instrumental processing for adequate demonstration. Thus, it differs from the classical reflex (macroreflex) in which the response is usually quite evident (for instance, patellar reflex, pupillary reflex, *etc*). without special instrumental assistance. In practice, microreflex responses are usually obtained by the statistical process of response averaging of electromyographic activity from the actively contracting muscle. These techniques have been found to reveal a large group of reflexes occurring at a "subliminal" level whose existence was formerly unsuspected. Some of the properties of the microreflex system are summarized in Fig. 1.

[1] Supported by U.S. Public Health Service Grants NS08961-02 and NS08962-02.

References p. 108

MICROREFLEXES

(1) *DEFINITION*   (a) *RESPONSE MUST BE SUBLIMINAL (NO MOVEMENT)*

                 (b) *RESPONSE IS REVEALED BY COMPUTER AVERAGING*

                 (c) *EFFECTOR (MUSCLE) MUST BE ACTIVE (TENSION)*

(2) *EVIDENCE FOR MYOGENIC ORIGIN*

   (A) *DISAPPEARANCE WITH*   (a) *CURARIZATION*

                             (b) *LOCAL NERVE BLOCK*

                             (c) *MUSCLE RELAXATION*

   (B) *APPEARANCE IN MUSCLE AREAS - e.g. ARM AND LEG*

   (C) *RECORDED FROM CLOSE BIPOLAR (CONCENTRIC) ELECTRODES*

(3) *OCCURRENCE PRESENT IN ANIMALS AND MAN*

Fig. 1. Summary of microreflex properties.

RECORDING TECHNIQUES

The salient points in recording of microreflexes are summarized in Fig. 2. The varieties
of stimuli employed so far are indicated to the left of the diagram. An important property of microreflexes is the relationship of their amplitude to the active tension existing
in the muscle from which the response is being sampled. In general, the size of the
response is linearly related to the active tension in the muscle so that the microreflex
disappears entirely from the totally relaxed muscle. This relationship requires that great
care be taken to standardize the degree of tension existing in muscles that are under-
going testing procedures for the measurement of the response. In general, the responses
are picked up from the muscle surface by standard EEG electrodes attached to the
overlying skin, and active tension in the muscle is controlled by a variety of mechanical
devices such as a pulley and loop attachment to the head, or a weight supported by the
arm, or in the case of muscles of expression by holding a required degree of contraction

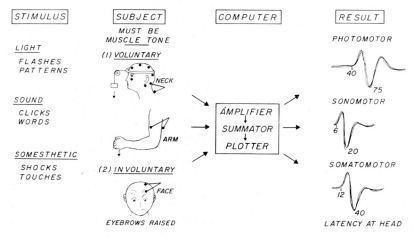

Fig. 2. Diagram of instrumental arrangements for the recording of microreflexes. Schematic responses with latency and peak values in milliseconds are shown on the right.

(such as eyebrow raising or teeth clenching) during the period of stimulation. The sampled EMG activity is then subjected to computer summation by a CAT or other computer system so that the responses that are time-locked to the stimulus can be extracted. The over-all frequency response of the recording system has usually been maintained at 2–100 c/sec. The computer response is usually graphed by an X-Y plotter and to the right of Fig. 2 the main sensory system responses with their latencies are shown. Note that the shortest latency response of about 6–8 msec (the sonomotor response) is recorded from the neck muscles (and elsewhere at greater latency). Shock stimuli applied to peripheral nerves will evoke an intermediate latency response of about 12 msec recorded from the scalp and inion regions (somatomotor responses). The response to flash stimuli (the photomotor response) has the longest latency of 40–70 msec and can be recorded for a total period of some 100–200 msec following the stimulus. Investigations have now been completed on four hundred and fifty-five normal subjects and one hundred and five patients with a variety of clinical disorders.

RESULTS

Photomotor response. Figure 3 illustrates a typical example of a photomotor micro-

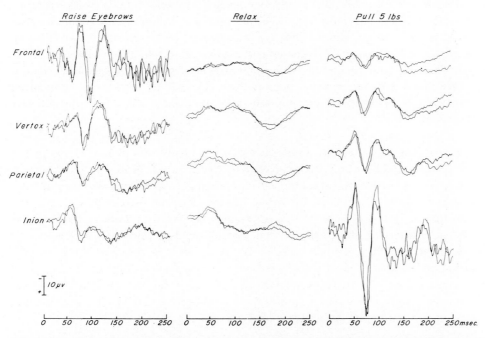

Fig. 3. Recording of the photomotor response in a normal subject. Center column, scalp muscles are relaxed and a visual evoked brain response is seen virtually free from myogenic components. The brain response is overwhelmed by myogenic components on the right and left sides when the microreflex is activated by steady tension (5 lbs. neck tension or raising eyebrows) during the period of photic stimulation (Grass photostimulator I = 8, 2 fl./sec). All derivations are referred to nose electrode, N = 100.

References p. 108

reflex recorded in a normal subject. In the center of the illustration note the recording of what is presumed to be a cortical evoked potential to photic stimuli without appreciable myogenic response. However, on the right, when tension is applied to the head, notice the appearance of a very large highly reliable response with a latency of about 50 msec and a main positive component at 75 msec. This is maximal in the region of muscle contraction (active tension). On the left side of the chart, the effect of shifting muscle tension to the frontalis muscle with raising of the eyebrows is illustrated. This results in the appearance of a highly reliable evoked response with a latency of about 50 msec but with components somewhat different from those evoked in the inion region. Note that the form of this reponse and the latency and over-all duration is quite similar to and overlaps in time that of the genuine evoked cortical response to photic stimulation. It can be obtained in virtually all normal subjects though there may be a hundredfold difference in amplitude between different members of the normal population. Thus, it is apparent that the microreflex can cause considerable difficulty in the interpretation of evoked potential data recorded from the scalp, particularly since myogenic responses are usually relatively smooth in contour and do not have the "spikey" characteristics that serve to distinguish muscle from genuine brain potentials in the primary EEG tracing. The photomotor response shows the approximately linear relation between active tension and response amplitude (Fig. 4) characteristic of all microreflexes. An example of a photomotor response recorded from a leg muscle is shown in Fig. 5. The amplitude of a photomotor response varies with the intensity of the stimulus and in a few subjects can be recorded down to visual threshold though the latency increases at these low levels and a large number of responses have to be summated to extract the response from the background. There is evidence that a genuine myogenic response can be obtained from visual stimulation with patterns though this kind of physiological stimulus has not yet been adequately investigated.

Somatomotor response. It was noted earlier that electrical stimulation of peripheral nerves in man could evoke a myogenic response (Cracco and Bickford 1966a, b) from the scalp and neck regions. An example of such a response to median nerve stimulation is shown in Fig. 6. Note that the latency of this response and its general form matches closely that of the somatosensory evoked response. The somatomotor response can be recorded with less facility in the normal population than other microreflexes. It is present in about 70% of normal subjects. While it is more widespread in topographic distribution than the somatosensory response, it may be very difficult to distinguish from genuine cortical activity, particularly in view of the fact that it is usually maximal contralateral to the side of nerve stimulation. It has been shown that this response can be obtained from the smaller nerves such as those which supply the digits.

Sonomotor response. The first microreflex discovered was an inion located response to click stimulation illustrated in Fig. 7. This response attracted immediate interest because of its extremely short latency (6–8 msec) and it was at first thought to be a response from the auditory cortex of the cerebellum. Further work, however, has

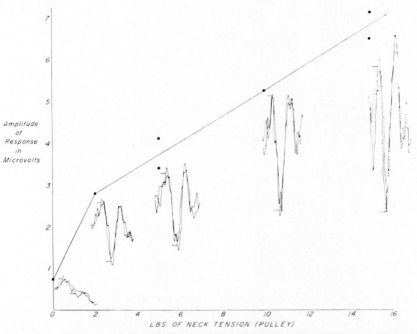

Fig. 4. Influence of neck tension on amplitude of photomotor response in a normal subject. Average of 100 inion responses to 2/sec photic stimulation. Measurements as indicated by markers on response samples. Weights applied by pulley. After initial sample relationship is approximately linear.

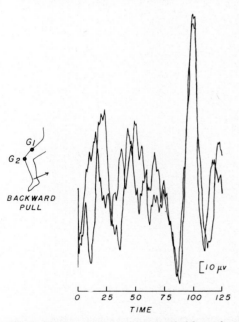

Fig. 5. Photomotor response recorded from the tensed quadriceps muscle. Average of 50 responses to 7.5/sec photic stimulation with eyes closed. Time scale in msec. Note response latency of about 60 msec. Stimulus intensity as in Fig. 3.

References p. 108

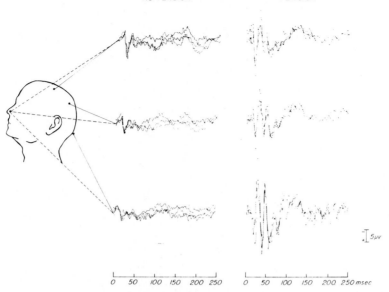

Fig. 6. Somatomotor response to maximal stimulation of the right median nerve; somatosensory response seen without neck tension has a latency of about 20 msec and is maximal over the contralateral somatosensory area (upper left tracing). With neck traction a larger, more complex and longer lasting response envelops the brain evoked potential (somatomotor response).

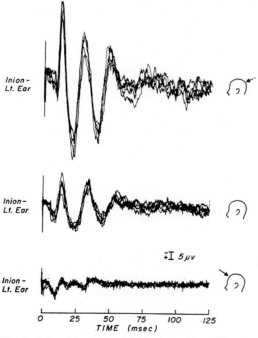

Fig. 7. Inion (sonomotor) response to binaural click stimulation in a normal subject. Five averages, each of 150 responses, superimposed. Intensity 120 dB. Upper traces with 5 lbs. neck tension; middle traces no tension with head erect; lower traces counter traction causing maximal relaxation of neck muscles, and virtual disappearance of inion response. Note short latency response with very low variance as indicated by close superimposition of successive traces.

proved that it is myogenic in origin as indicated by its virtual disappearance when the neck muscles are relaxed as in the lower part of Fig. 7. In the course of these investigations, a similar latency response was recorded more laterally and particularly behind the pinna in normal subjects. It was soon recognized that this response was the same as that which had been recorded by Kiang *et al.* (1963) who apparently were in some doubt as to whether this was an intracranial or extracranial response. The post-auricular response is illustrated in Fig. 8 which also proves its myogenic nature by showing that it can be suppressed by blocking (with local anesthesia) the small branch of the facial nerve that supplies the post-auricular muscles. Likewise, the response can be simulated by stimulation of the nerve after recovery of the block (Fig. 8).

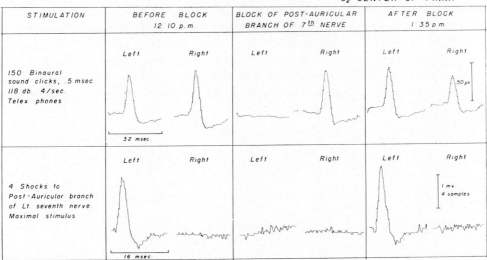

Fig. 8. Effect of nerve block and nerve stimulation on post-auricular response, recorded from post-auricular electrode referred to center of pinna. Response is of simpler contour than the inion response. Block of left post-auricular nerve eliminates response (upper row) which subsequently recovers. Lower row shows a simulation of the response produced by nerve stimulation with disappearance of the simulated response after nerve block with subsequent recovery.

Further investigation of the inion sonomotor response has shown it to have some unexpected and interesting properties. For instance, the intensity-response relationship for click stimuli is quite unusual in shape for a sensory receptor insofar as there is evidence of increasing sensitivity up to an allowable intensity of sound stimulation and furthermore, that in many normal subjects the response disappears at relatively high sound levels of about 90–110 dB (Fig. 9). Investigations in patients with cochlear and vestibular nerve lesions has further demonstrated that the receptor involved in the inion response does not appear to be the cochlea since the response may be present in a deaf ear, if the vestibular system is intact (Fig. 10). In further investigations of the vestibular system in relation to this response, Townsend and Cody (1971) have shown that the response is probably originating from the saccular part of the vestibular apparatus.

References p. 108

Thus it appears that the sonomotor inion response is likely to provide a significant clinical test of saccular function in the human, though further investigation is required before the validity of this test can be firmly established.

An interesting recent observation which relates to the above problem is a finding illustrated in Fig. 11 which has been obtained in two normal subjects. The inion and post-auricular responses are recorded to a high intensity click stimulus which is eventually masked to inaudibility by random noise fed to the same ear. In some, but not all subjects a clearly defined inion response can still be obtained even though the click stimulus has become inaudible. It is interesting that under these circumstances the post-auricular response which appears to originate from the cochlea is entirely suppressed. Thus, the masking tone serves to differentiate between the two types of receptors. The neuronal mechanism of this rather unexpected finding is being investigated. It is interesting, however, that this experiment represents an input and output from the central nervous system that has occurred at a subliminal level without conscious recognition.

There is a trend in evoked potential work in the human to use more physiological and often more sophisticated stimuli to activate the central processing mechanisms. This type of approach can also be taken with the microreflex and Fig. 12 illustrates an example in which a myogenic response from the post-auricular region is evoked by a

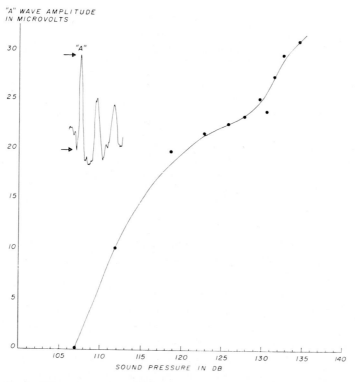

Fig. 9. Effect of sound intensity on amplitude of inion sonomotor response in a normal subject with 23 lbs. neck traction. Measurements made on response as indicated by arrows. In this subject the response was not obtainable below a threshold of 107 dB.

word rather than a crude and meaningless click or tone burst stimulus. This effect is analogous to that already mentioned for the photomotor system in which pattern stimuli can become an adequate input for the microreflex system.

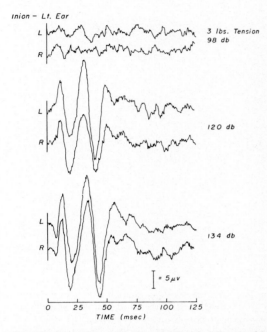

Fig. 10. Recording of inion response in 18-year-old patient with total hearing loss in the right ear (labyrinths normal). Monaural stimulation of left (*L*) and right (*R*) ears at increasing dB levels. Note equal response in spite of deafness in right ear indicating a probable vestibular origin for the response. Separate evidence indicates that the sonomotor response cannot be initiated from the opposite ear (no crossover).

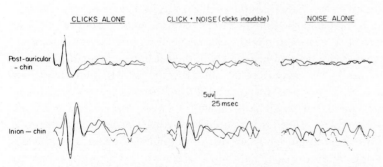

Fig. 11. Effect of a masking sound on post-auricular and inion responses in normal subject with 6 lbs. inion tension. Left column monaural stimulation at 12 dB with clicks alone. Center column random noise is added (acoustic mixing) until clicks are inaudible. This suppresses the post-auricular response but leaves the inion response only slightly reduced. Control for random noise alone on the right.

References p. 108

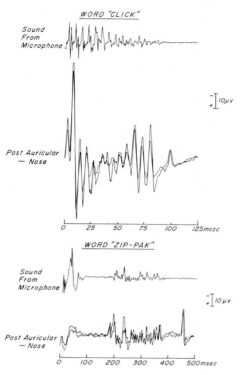

Fig. 12. Stimulation with words "click" and "zip-pak". Words were recorded on a tape loop. Sound from tape was summated (top traces) to indicate approximate form of the word stimulus. Sound level approximately 110 dB. Note the highly reliable myogenic responses obtained (average of 150).

ANIMAL OBSERVATIONS

The work of Kern *et al.* (1969) has indicated the feasibility of recording myogenic responses in the rat and guinea pig that seem to parallel some of the microreflex responses noted in the human. However, the responses investigated by the above workers have been found to originate from the cochlear receptors and so are analogous to the post-auricular response in the human rather than the inion response. Another interesting response to click stimulation in the cat has been reported by Lee and Bickford (1967). This response can be obtained widely in the cat but is maximal in the neck muscles and is produced by click stimuli of 20–100 dB (Fig. 13). The remarkable feature of this response is its latency and the fact that it is not always present in members of the cat population. The extremely short latency of 2.5 msec has raised some questions as to whether a complete reflex circuit could be involved or whether this represents some kind of artifactual situation. There seems no doubt, however, that this is a genuine microreflex and interesting artifact control is shown in Fig. 14 in which the microreflex is suppresssed by barbiturate, leaving the evoked cortical response relatively unaffected. It is not yet known whether this reflex arises from the cochlear or vestibular receptor of the cat's inner ear mechanism.

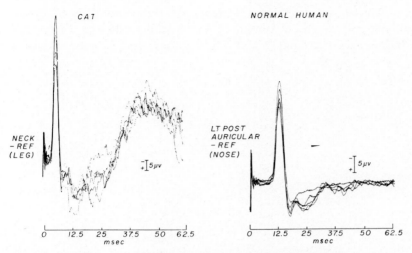

Fig. 13. Comparison of post-auricular microreflex recorded from man and from cat. Animal un-anesthetized, semirestrained, neck electrode placed as shown in Figure 14, 5 averages each of 400 responses, to 4/sec clicks at 110 dB. Normal human subject, 5 averages each 150 responses to 7.5/sec clicks at 134 dB.

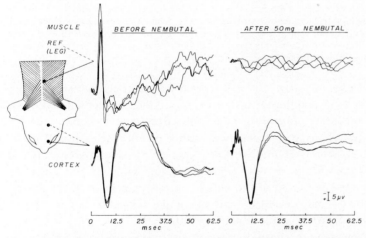

Fig. 14. Suppression of the post-auricular response in the cat by anesthesia. The cortical evoked re-sponse (lower traces) are relatively unaffected. Average of 500 responses, 3 runs, 110 dB click.

CLINICAL APPLICATION FOR LESION LOCALIZATION

The system of microreflexes already described represents a large variety of reflex pathways involving a wide spectrum of central nervous system structures. Thus, they add greatly to the repertoire of tests already available to the neurologist through the classical macroreflex systems (patella, pupil, *etc.*). Since microreflex tests can be carried out easily and quickly (provided that an averager system is available), they offer an

References p. 108

important new tool in the clinical area. For instance, the sonomotor response can be tested and the result graphed in two minutes. (With a stimulus rate of 7.5/sec, 150 responses can be summated in about 21 sec). Fig. 15 illustrates a patient in whom a

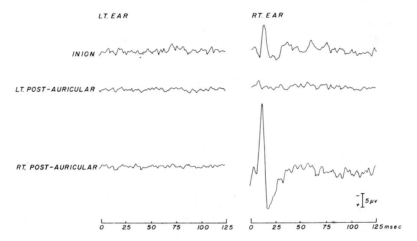

Fig. 15. Changes in sonomotor responses (inion and post-auricular) in a patient with a pontine tumor. Age 23 years. Paralysis of left 6th, 7th and 8th cranial nerves. Left column, left ear stimulated (134 dB), shows no response because input is blocked by lesion in 8th nerve. Right column, right ear stimulated, shows a normal inion response and right post-auricular response but the left post-auricular response is suppressed due to the lesion of the left facial nerve. This illustrates the use of microreflexes to locate lesions in both input and output pathways.

pontine lesion had blocked a variety of reflex input and output pathways with a resulting elimination of some sonomotor responses. One difficulty encountered in the clinical application of these reflex tests is their dependence on the level of active tension in the muscles under test. Thus, at present, they cannot be effectively applied in the uncooperative, confused, or unconscious patient. However, the testing procedure can be modified so that stimuli are given only when a required range of EMG activity (determined by computer integration of the muscle output) is present in the muscle under test. This method is being developed and may make clinical testing feasible in the absence of active cooperation on the part of the patient.

In addition to blocking of microreflexes by a lesion, the inverse phenomenon, that of facilitation may be observed. This occurs in various forms of myoclonus and raises the question in any particular case as to whether the normal microreflex pathway or some pathologic routing of the discharge is occurring. A useful criterion here is the latency of the myoclonic response and the degree to which it matches the microreflex latency measurements made in the normal subject. So far, such comparisons have been made only for the stimulus-sensitive myoclonus of the photic variety. Thus, Broughton *et al.* (1967) have reported that in some cases of photomyoclonus the latency of the response in the face (50 msec) does approximate that of the photomotor response. In these cases a pathological sensitivity of the photomotor pathway appears to be a valid explanation. An example from one of our patients with a comparison to a normal subject is shown in Fig. 16. However, it is very clear that other forms of photomyoclonus occur in which the photomotor pathway cannot be implicated. This is particularly the case in the photic sensitivity observed in a variety of degenerative conditions (e.g. Jakob-Creutzfeldt disease) which frequently show longer latencies and which are further characterized by large fluctuations in latency from one stimulus to another.

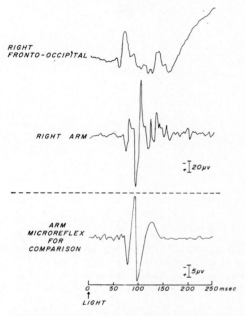

Fig. 16. Myoclonic response (average of 25) to light in a photosensitive 49-year-old epileptic patient. It illustrates a good latency match between a photomotor response recorded in the arm of a normal subject (bottom trace) and the single response of the epileptic patient to a flash of light. The accompanying cortical response is shown in the top trace.

PHYSIOLOGIC MECHANISMS OPERATIVE IN MICROREFLEXES

Some of the problems of the receptor mechanisms in microreflexes have already been discussed and here we will take up those concerned with the synthesis of the electrical discharge recorded from the muscle surface in microreflex observations. In considering the origin of these discharges, it is evident from Fig. 17 that little is gained by examining the individual surface potentials from which the average is derived. In these it is rarely possible to recognize any individual component from which the averaged contour is derived indicating how remarkably effective this form of processing is in revealing the hidden time-locked elements of the discharge. When the muscle is searched with a needle electrode for evidence of the unit generators there is a variety of findings depending on the position of the tip in relation to the motor unit, whether the latter is entrained by the stimulus, and whether individual or summated data are reviewed. An example of the findings is shown in Fig. 18. Note the simplicity of the surface sum-

References p. 108

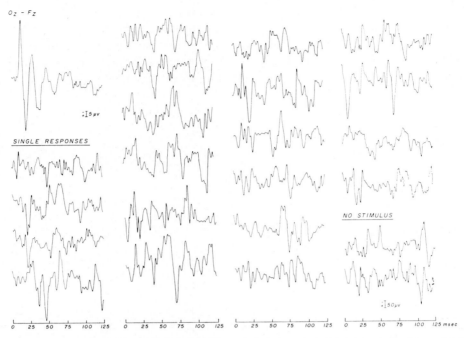

Fig. 17. Components of the inion responses to click stimulation in a normal subject with 10 lbs. tension. The form of the summated inion response is shown at upper left. The single responses show 20 of the 150 responses from which the summation was made. Note that it is difficult to recognize the features of the summated response in any one of the individual responses. Two no stimulus sweeps are shown in the right lower corner.

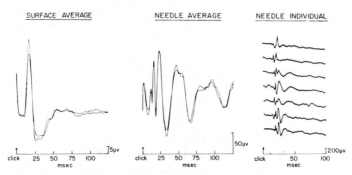

Fig. 18. Comparison of post-auricular responses to click stimulation (recorded from left post-auricular electrode referred to chin, in relaxed normal subject) with different recording methods. *Left*: average from surface electrode; *middle*: average made from needle electrode; *right*: a series of single sweeps recorded from a needle electrode within the muscle.

mated data as compared to the summated data from a responding unit or that obtained from single sweeps without summation. It should be noted that the commonest finding from needle exploration of a muscle is to observe little or no relationship between needle-derived, single or summated activity and that summated from the surface electrode. This indicates that only a small proportion of the units are entrained to follow the stimulus. Complexities are also caused by the position of the needle tip in relation to the rest of the fiber (since this is the region which shows initial negativity in relation to other regions), by pick up of more than one unit, and by latency differences in discharge between different fibers within the motor unit.

The functional significance of the microreflex system remains obscure. There has been a suggestion that it functions as a tension setting (priming) device to prepare the muscle for maximal response to a startle stimulus. At least in the case of the sonomotor pathways this information would reach the muscle well ahead of the startle response. Thus in the neck muscles sonomotor information arrives about 6–8 msec following a stimulus whereas the startle movement occurs at about 50 msec. This raises the further question of whether the gamma efferent system is involved in generating the microreflex response. Unfortunately at present there is no evidence available to answer this question.

CONCLUSION

The properties of microreflexes (summarized in Fig. 1) appear consistent enough to justify the designation of a system with sonomotor, photomotor and somatomotor components. Their applications in various disciplines may be summarized as follows: to the electroencephalographer they pose difficult problems in differentiation from evoked potentials that can only be solved by special testing procedures. For the neurologist there are a large variety of clinical applications both as a new test of vestibular function (saccule) and in their ability to demonstrate lesions by blocking and facilitatory effects within the CNS. To the neuropharmacologist the system is of considerable interest because of the sensitivity of microreflexes to drug action. Thus they are suppressed early by anesthetics and by diazepam and markedly accentuated by some convulsants (pentylenetetrazol). To the psychologist the great variability of these responses in the normal population suggests that some individuals may possess a facilitated pathway from receptor to muscle, a difference in basic response mechanism that might relate to personality variables such as tension, anxiety, *etc*. Likewise there should be an interesting field for investigation in the various types of psychosis and anxiety reactions.

In these varied endeavors the existence of several animal models that exhibit at least some of the system properties will assist in the study of some basic mechanisms that have not yet received adequate attention.

ACKNOWLEDGEMENTS

This acknowledges valued assistance in various phases of this work from Dr. Cody, Dr. Jacobson and Miss Lee Stewart.

References p. 108

REFERENCES

BICKFORD, R. G. Nature of computer averaged evoked potentials in man. *Fed. Proc.*, **1963**, *22*: 678.

BICKFORD, R. G. Properties of the photomotor response system. *Electroenceph. clin. Neurophysiol.*, **1964**a, *17*: 456.

BICKFORD, R. G. The interaction of averaged multisensory responses recorded at the inion. *Electroenceph. clin. Neurophysiol.*, **1964**b, *17*: 713.

BICKFORD, R. G. Human "microreflexes" revealed by computer analysis. *Neurology (Minneap.)*, **1966**a, *16*: 302.

BICKFORD, R. G. Microreflex contamination of sensory (visual) evoked scalp potentials in man. *Fed. Proc.*, **1966**b, *25*: 574.

BICKFORD, R. G. Effect of facial expression on the averaged evoked response to light in man. *Electroenceph. clin. Neurophysiol.*, **1967**, *23*: 78–79.

BICKFORD, R. G. and KLASS, D. W. Sensory precipitation and reflex mechanisms. In H. H. JASPER, A. A. WARD and A. POPE (EDS.), *Basic mechanisms of the epilepsies*. Little, Brown, Boston, **1969**: 543.

BICKFORD, R. G., JACOBSON, J. L. and CODY, D. T. R. Opportunities and pitfalls in the processing of neuroelectric data: observations on averaged evoked potentials recorded from the scalp in man. *Proc. 5th IBM Med. Symp.*, **1963**a: 401–418.

BICKFORD, R. G., JACOBSON, J. L. and CODY, D. T. R. Nature of evoked potentials to sound and other stimuli in man. *Ann. N. Y. Acad. Sci.*, **1964**a, *112*: 204–223.

BICKFORD, R. G., JACOBSON, J. L., CODY, D. T. R. and LAMBERT, E. H. Fast motor systems in man: physiopathology of the sonomotor response. *Trans. Amer. Neurol. Ass.*, **1964**b, *89*: 56–58.

BICKFORD, R. G., JACOBSON, J. L. and GALBRAITH, R. F. A new audiomotor system in man. *Electroenceph. clin. Neurophysiol.*, **1963**b, *15*: 922.

BICKFORD, R. G., SPEHLMANN, C. R. F., JACOBSON, J. L. and GALBRAITH, R. F. Application of response averaging in neurology. *Neurology (Minneap)*, **1963**c, *13*: 354.

BROUGHTON, R., MEIER-EWERT, K. and EBE, M. Evoked visual, somatosensory, myogenic, oculogenic and electroretinographic potentials of photosensitive epileptic patients and normal control subjects. *Electroenceph. clin. Neurophysiol.*, **1967**, *23*: 492 P.

CODY, D. T. R. and BICKFORD, R. G. Cortical audiometry: an objective method of evaluating auditory acuity in man. *Proc. Mayo Clin.*, **1965**, *40*: 273–287.

CODY, D. T. R., GUTRECHT, J. A. and BICKFORD, R. G. Averaged evoked potentials to sound stimulation in guinea pigs. *Fed. Proc.*, **1965**, *24*: 206.

CODY, D. T. R., JACOBSON, J. L., WALKER, J. C. and BICKFORD, R. G. Averaged evoked myogenic and cortical potentials to sound in man. *Ann. Otol. (St. Louis)*, **1964**, *73*: 763–778.

CRACCO, R. Q. and BICKFORD, R. G. Comparison of evoked somatosensory and somatomotor responses in man. *Electroenceph. clin. Neurophysiol.*, **1966**a, *21*: 412 P.

CRACCO, R. Q. and BICKFORD, R. G. The somatomotor response to median nerve stimulation in man. *Electroenceph. clin. Neurophysiol.*, **1966**b, *20*: 97 P.

JACOBSON, J. L., CODY, D. T. R., LAMBERT, E. H. and BICKFORD, R. G. Physiological properties of the postauricular response (sonomotor) in man. *Physiologist*, **1964**a, *7*: 167.

JACOBSON, J. L., LAMBERT, E. H. and BICKFORD, R. G. Nature of the averaged auricular response to sound stimulation in man. *Electroenceph. clin. Neurophysiol.*, **1964**b, *17*: 609 P.

KERN, E. B., CODY, D. T. R. and BICKFORD, R. G. Averaged evoked potentials to auditory stimuli recorded from dural electrodes in guinea pigs. *Arch. Otolaryng.*, **1969**, *90*: 315–325.

KIANG, N. Y-S., CRIST, A. H., FRENCH, M. A. and EDWARDS, A. G. Postauricular electric response to acoustic stimuli in humans. In *Quarterly progress report, Research Lab. Electronics*. M. I. T., Boston, **1963**: 218–225.

LEE, N. and BICKFORD, R. G. Click evoked microreflex and cortical potentials in the cat. *Electroenceph. clin. Neurophysiol.*, **1967**, *23*: 492 P.

TOWNSEND, C. L. and CODY, D. T. R. The averaged inion response evoked by acoustic stimulation: its relation to the saccule. *Ann. Otol. (St. Louis)*, **1971**, *80*: 121–132.

Some New Experiments on Cerebellar Motor Control[1]

VERNON B. BROOKS[2]

Department of Physiology, New York Medical College, New York, N.Y. 10029 (U.S.A.)

Today we are honouring Herbert Jasper who can look back from the vantage point of current active research to a lifetime of study, in which he has given us many basic insights that form the foundation of much of our understanding of central nervous function. This is especially true of the sensorimotor system, which has long been a topic of primary interest in Montreal. Concern about the controls of input and output flowed quite naturally down the hill of University Street from the Neurological Institute to the Physiology Department where I worked from 1952 to 1956. Fascination with this topic captured me eventually in 1958, when I began research on input to the cat's motor cortex at the Rockefeller Institute. This work finally revealed that some information from skin and joints was organized somatotopically in columns of cells in motor cortex, providing a framework for incoming convergence (Welt *et al.* 1967). The related work by Asanuma and Sakata (1967) and Asanuma *et al.* (1968) linked the pyramidal output from cell colonies in such columns to particular spinal motor nuclei, capable of tensing the muscles that move the limb when it is in the path of relevant skin stimuli. This led to the concept of columnar, minimal input–output building blocks of motor cortex, which are thought to participate in voluntary movements even though their simplest action is only a stereotyped positive feedback. Versatility is presumably introduced through various forms of higher control from other parts of the cortex, the cerebellum and other structures (Brooks 1969). In the pursuit of higher control mechanisms for motor cortex, we have lately turned to the study of cerebellar function. It is not clear to what extent the cerebellum acts in initiation, as opposed to feedback control, of cortically mediated movements (Evarts and Thach 1969). It is clear, however, that the cerebellum is essential to normal motion: when it is damaged we can lose control over the force, velocity and displacement of voluntary movement (Holmes 1939). Force is the basic parameter of cerebral motor control: it reflects the degrees of activation of spinal motor centers, at the minimal level presumably as output of cortical columns. Velocity is related inescapably to force in most types of movements, and displacement is the result of application of force. We have focussed our attention on the lateral aspect of the cerebellar hemispheres, because they exert control on motor cortex, mostly through the dentate outflow *via* the ventrolateral nucleus. The intermediate aspects act more directly on the spinal cord,

[1] Supported in part by U.S. Public Health Service Research and Training Grants NB-05508 and NB-05544 and Grant GB-8018 from the National Science Foundation.
[2] Present address: Department of Physiology, University of Western Ontario, London 72, Canada.

References p. 116

mostly through outflow from n. interpositus (IP) *via* the red nucleus. Thus dentate is thought to be most important for voluntary movements, while IP may be more relevant for reflex adjustments and posture. Both nuclei receive information from skin, joints and muscles, paralleling input to motor cortex (Eccles 1969; Evarts and Thach 1969).

At this time I would like to describe briefly some new experiments on cerebellar control of movement that arose from our interest in the motor cortex. This work has been carried out during the past 3 years at the New York Medical College, in various associations with Drs. Kozlovskaya, Horvath, Atkin, Uno and Fuller. We have studied the effects of temporary cerebellar dysfunction on motor control through the use of reversible, local cooling of the dentate and IP nuclei in *Cebus* monkeys. The cooling technique was introduced to us by Dr. Sharpless, and has been described by Byck and Jennings (1969). Cooling sheaths were implanted stereotaxically, together with thermocouples and electrodes. In an initial experiment, we studied free-reaching "complex" movements, as Holmes (1939) called them. The animal had to reach for and to press two bars alternately for grape juice reinforcement (Horvath *et al.* 1970). Cooling of the dentate nucleus to 20–10°C brought on several signs of cerebellar disease on the ipsilateral side: the rate of performance slowed, with concurrent increase of incorrect

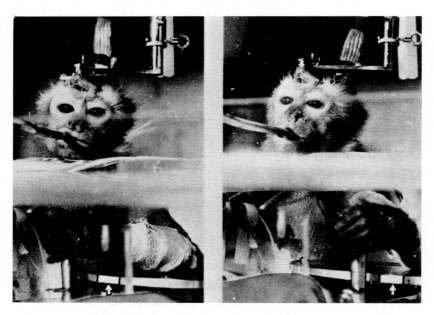

Fig. 1. Experimental arrangement. Frontal views of monkey No. 4 sitting in the experimental chair and holding handle of manipulandum; elbow is flexed in the left picture and extended in the right. Target areas are indicated by white boxes and arrows. Towel sleeve around arm covers skin EMG electrodes. The towel jacket around the trunk restrains monkey. An opaque platform obstructing the animal's vision of the field of motion is seen between hand and head. The fluid reward tube is seen in front of his mouth. Animal's head is held by an adjustable clamp attached to studs embedded in skull. Leads from implanted electrodes in brachium conjunctivum, dentate and interpositus nuclei can be seen emerging from a plug implanted in the skull. (From: Kozlovskaya, I., Atkin, A., Horvath, F., Uno, M. and Brooks, V. B., 1968, unpublished data.)

alternations. The reaching phases to a point distant in space lengthened particularly, and muscular coordination worsened. Movements decomposed into successive components, and oscillatory searching occurred.

Subsequently, more exact tests were made with "simple" movements (Holmes 1939) in which five chronically implanted animals were trained to execute a step-tracking task with the arm ipsilateral to the cooled nucleus. The task, which primarily involved movement about the elbow joint, required accuracy of movements without prescribing force or velocity. The monkeys were trained to move a handle that pivoted freely, without opposing forces, in a horizontal arc about the elbow, back and forth between two target zones. The movement swept through approximately 35–50° and had to stop accurately in each target zone of 10–15° width for about 1.0 sec. After holding the handle in the target for the required time, the monkey had to return the handle to the alternate target. Fig. 1 shows a monkey in the chair, with the operant arm in the flexion target (left photograph) and in the extension target (right). The elbow was firmly supported near the level of shoulder height to allow forearm movement about the elbow joint to be carried out mainly by biceps and triceps muscles. The targets, indicated by white arrows in the pictures, were not bounded by mechanical stops, but the animal learned their positions through auditory cues: an "on-target tone" sounded when the handle was in the target. Vision of the task area was blocked. When the animals had successfully reached and stayed in the correct alternate targets, they were rewarded with juice. Training periods of the animals could be shortened from months to weeks by letting them work in their cages for their daily water. Fig. 2 illustrates the "self-service" apparatus used for successively harder tasks that prepared them for daily work sessions in the laboratory.

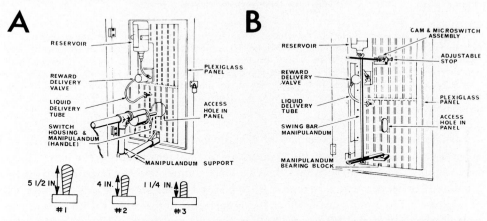

Fig. 2. Devices used for pretraining monkeys in their cages. *A.* Single-lever manipulandum for initial phase of pretraining: monkey can reach handle through access hole in transparent plastic cage-front panel. Each time monkey pushes handle he receives a squirt of water from mouthpiece mounted on panel. # *1, 2, 3* (bottom of sketch): as training progressed, handles of successively shorter lengths (#*2, 3*) were substituted for the long handle (#*1*) used at the start. *B.* Alternate position-change manipulandum for second phase of pretraining. Monkey can reach vertical bar through access hole in transparent plastic cage-front panel. If he moves bar horizontally back and forth through an arc from stop to stop, remaining against each stop for a preset required time, he receives a squirt of water each time. (From: Atkin, A., Horvath, F., Kozlovskaya, I. and Brooks, V.B., 1968, unpublished data.)

References p. 116

Our measurements were made of derivatives of force, namely velocity and displacement, because the animals could move the handle at their own speeds. Well-trained monkeys performed the movements either in "fast", continuous, smooth motions, or in "slow", stepwise discontinuous motions. The monkeys shifted from continuous fast to discontinuous slow movements when their routine was disturbed by any one of many factors. Durations of fast movements were tightly clustered about a mean of about 0.5 sec. Durations of slow movements, in contrast, were more widely dispersed as their numbers of constituent steps was variable (Kozlovskaya *et al.* 1970b). A sample record in Fig. 3 shows the relations of the targets and the outer mechanical stops in a typical run, where the animal used slow movements. The discontinuities of displacement are seen more clearly in the velocity record below.

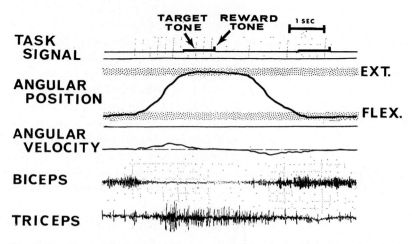

Fig. 3. Sample record of a control movement. Angular position is read out from the potentiometer mounted on the axis of the manipulandum handle. The stipled target zones are 10° of arc in width, and separated by 40°. Mechanical stops are 15° further, indicated by horizontal lines, but not labelled. Angular velocity is read out as the derivation of angular position. Note clear alternation of biceps and triceps activity in EMG traces. Task signal line at the top indicates "target" and "reward" tones. (Monkey 4L.) (From: Kozlovskaya, I., Atkin, A., Horvath, F., Uno, M. and Brooks V.B., 1969, unpublished data.)

Task performance, and the effects of dentate cooling, are explained most easily by inspection of a sample record. Fig. 4 illustrates control movements in the upper trace, carried out as fast extensions and flexions. This animal had not experienced many changes of the experimental regime. The upper and lower sets of traces compare actions separated by 1 min, during which the temperature of the probe sheath tip near the rostrolateral end of the dentate nucleus was lowered to 10 °C. Regular alternations during controls are contrasted with irregular, dysmetric movements during dentate cooling. These trials were easy, since the target zones were wide and separated only by a short distance. The regular rhythmical record begins with a successful stay in the flexor (lower) target, as signalled by the reward tone (downward signal marker). Extension-1 terminated within the extension target, but the monkey slightly anticipated the end of the 0.7 sec required time of stay within the target and left it with slow flexion-

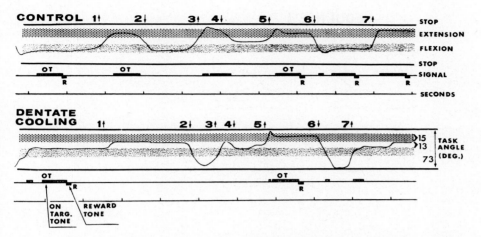

Fig. 4. Movement patterns before and during cooling of the dentate nucleus. Upper set of records: control run recorded immediately before start of cooling. Lower set of records: movements recorded while probe tip temperature near rostroventral end of dentate was at 10°C, recorded 1 min after start of cooling. Upward (↑) deflections show extensions of the forearm and downward (↓) deflections show flexions. Each such movement is numbered. The shaded bands show the extension and flexion target zones, each of 15° width. Distance between targets was 13° of arc, as labelled at right of lower set of records. Heavy boundary lines indicate position of mechanical stops (limiting the maximum range of movement), distance between which corresponded to 73° of arc. All task angles within this total range are marked on the right margin of the lower set of records. Upward markers indicate target-tone (*OT*) when the handle was in the correct target, and downward markers indicate reward-tones, after the lever had been held in the target continuously for 0.7 sec. (Monkey # 3.) (From: Kozlovskaya, I., Atkin, A., Horvath, F. and Brooks, V. B., 1968, unpublished data.)

2 before receiving a reward tone. (Note absence of *R* signal at end of *OT* signal after extension-1.) The subsequent extension-3 overshot the target slightly. This was quickly corrected, but flexion-4 followed too soon thereafter, again thwarting a reward. The monkey undershot the flexion target in flexion-4, but held the handle anyway in this wrong position for about the correct time. Extension-5 finally brought success, as did subsequent flexion-6 and extension-7, giving a score of 4 out of 8 in this particular 10-sec sequence. In the lower record there is wild over- and undershooting, resulting in half the successes reached in the control, also with 7 target approaches per 10-sec period. The undershot extension-1 movement was held for an abnormally long time, followed by an overshoot in the flexion-2 movement. Since the extension-1 movement had not ended in success, the extension target remained the correct target, so that no target tone occurred as the monkey passed through the flexion target during flexion-2 and the following extension-3 and flexion-4 movements. The extension-3 again undershot, as did the subsequent flexion-4. Success was finally reached with extension-5, although it had to be quickly corrected for initial overshoot. Flexion-6 was marked by extreme overshooting, and the corrective extension-7 movement was also unsuccessful. This trial with fast movements reveals dysmetria, irregularity and reduced success.

In *Sequence I* of Fig. 5 cooling of the probe sheath tip near the dentate nucleus to 10°C caused another monkey to shift from regular, successful control alternations to

References p. 116

SEQUENCE 1

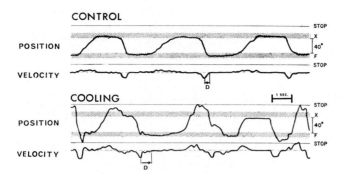

SEQUENCE 2

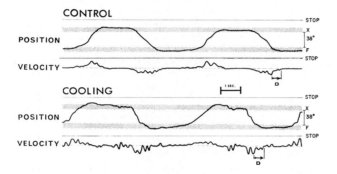

Fig. 5. Upper set of records in each sequence taken during a control run, and lower set during cooling of the rostral tip of the dentate nucleus to near 10 °C. Target zones are stipled: X extension up, and F flexion down. Intertarget distance marked. Deceleration times are marked D under velocity traces. (Monkey 4L.) (From: Kozlovskaya, I., Atkin, A., Horvath, F., Uno, M. and Brooks, V.B., 1969, unpublished data.)

dysmetric movements, overshooting the targets more than before. Our velocity records show that these errors of displacement were accompanied by excessive peak values and fluctuations of velocity. This was true for movements in either direction, which were slow extensions and fast flexions in the control period. (This animal had already experienced a number of experimental variations.) *Sequence 2*, recorded after a further 2 months of experiments with this animal, illustrates control and cooling runs characteristic of "experienced" animals. The animal now used slow movements in extensions and flexions in control, and it compensated for dysmetria by reaching both targets correctly with slow movements. Yet peak velocity fluctuations were still greater during dentate cooling than in controls (Brooks *et al.* 1969; Kozlovskaya *et al.* 1969). Peak velocities increased for fast movements through increases of acceleration, which became briefer than in normal movements. At the same time decelerations lengthened, (see Fig. 5. *Sequence 1* "D" marked below velocity traces of flexions), and for slow movements became tremorously fluctuating (see *Sequence 2*). The essential result obtained in our experiments with unopposed movements was the demonstration that dentate cooling caused reversible loss of velocity control, with increase of velocity fluctuations.

The effects of dentate cooling became more pronounced as the temperature was lowered progressively from 20 °C, to 10 °C, to 5 °C in the same, or in different trials. Was this due to involvement of other nearby structures? Direct tests showed that the effects produced by dentate cooling were specific to the dentate nucleus. Analogous local cooling of IP, located only a few millimeters medially, did not necessarily lead to this loss of velocity control or to hypermetria (Uno *et al*. 1971). While dentate cooling produced large changes in voluntary movements and IP cooling did not, IP cooling did produce larger changes than dentate cooling in reflex adjustments of a flexor jerk superimposed on voluntary movements (Brooks *et al*. 1970). This result fits the expected function of IP on spinal mechanisms.

Finally, let us return to the theme that led us into this research: the relationship between processing of peripheral sensory input from the moving limb and the nature of cerebellar control of voluntary movement. What guidance was used by the monkeys for arm movements in the tracking task? Was the information from receptors in the limb itself more important than external information such as auditory cues? The monkeys demonstrated this to be true by learning to work accurately without target tones through the use of slow discontinuous movements. Moreover, during dentate cooling the animals became more dependent on external clues: they could not perform the task without target tones. Corroboration came from another set of experiments in which the target tone was not withheld, but instead it was falsely presented at different positions between the correct target zones. In normal movements, spurious insertion of false target signals did not produce any significant changes in the main parts of ongoing movements. During dentate cooling, however, the vulnerability to false signals increased: now their insertion caused significant alterations in larger parts of the movements (Kozlovskaya *et al*. 1970a). Thus, input from the operant limb seems critical for dentate function in motor control. The internal guidance system which serves well enough normally, seems to become inadequate during dentate cooling. The fault is not likely an afferent loss, since patients with cerebellar lesions are said to have normal recognition of joint position (De Jong 1958). Instead, the fault appears to depend upon abnormal processing of such information from the moving limb.

Holmes summarized his view of cerebellar dysfunction, derived from clinical observations, in the Hughlings Jackson Memorial Lecture in 1938, published in 1939, as follows: "If a single movement is studied, such as flexion or extension of a single finger, or of the forearm at the elbow, while the rest of the limb is supported or fixed, the most prominent abnormalities are due to disturbances in its rate." Our experiments have led us to the same conclusion, and they lend credence to the supposition that the lateral cerebellum may function as an important timing device for movements, and presumably for the motor cortex.

References p. 116

SUMMARY

Brief local cooling of monkeys' dentate nucleus causes temporary symptoms of ip-silateral cerebellar disease. "Complex" free reaching movements become slowed, dyscoordinated and oscillatory, quick alternation between two targets fails and the movements become decomposed. "Simple" tracking task movements of guiding a handle, freely moving without opposing forces between alternate targets, initially undergo loss of position and velocity control. After compensation of the dysmetria, loss of velocity control remains, revealed through excessive velocity fluctuations. These effects are specific for dentate dysfunction as they are not necessarily obtained by cooling the interposed nuclei.

REFERENCES

ASANUMA, H. and SAKATA, H. Functional organization of a cortical efferent system examined with focal depth stimulation in cats. *J. Neurophysiol.*, **1967**, *30*: 35–54.
ASANUMA, H., STONEY, S.D. and ABZUG, C. Relationship between afferent input and motor outflow in cat motorsensory cortex. *J. Neurophysiol.*, **1968**, *31*: 670–681.
BROOKS, V.B. Information processing in motorsensory cortex. In K.N. LEIBOVIC (ED.), *Information processing in the nervous system*. Springer-Verlag, New York, **1969**: 231–243.
BROOKS, V.B., ATKIN, A., KOZLOVSKAYA, I. and UNO, M. Motor effects from interposed nuclei. *Physiologist*, **1970**, *13*: 157.
BROOKS, V.B., HORVATH, F., ATKIN, A., KOZLOVSKAYA, I. and UNO, M. Reversible changes in volun-tary movement during cooling of a subcerebellar nucleus. *Fed. Proc.*, **1969**, *28*: 396.
BYCK, R. and JENNINGS JR., C.B. Methods for long term local cooling of the brain in unrestrained animals. *Amer. J. appl. Physiol.*, **1969**, *27*: 144–148.
DE JONG, R.N. *The neurologic examination, 2nd edition*. Hoeber-Harper, New York, **1958**, 411 p.
ECCLES, J.C. The dynamic loop hypothesis of movement control. In K.N. LEIBOVIC (ED.), *Information processing in the nervous system*. Springer-Verlag, New York, **1969**, 245–269.
EVARTS, E.V. and THACH, W.T. Motor mechanisms of the CNS: cerebro-cerebellar interrelations. *Ann. Rev. Physiol.*, **1969**, *31*: 451–498.
HOLMES, G. The cerebellum of man. *Brain*, **1939**, *62*: 1–30.
HORVATH, F., ATKIN, A., KOZLOVSKAYA, I., FULLER, D.R.G. and BROOKS, V.B. Effects of cooling the dentate nucleus on alternating bar-pressing performance in monkey. *Int. J. Neurol. (Montevideo)*, **1970**, *7*: 252–270.
KOZLOVSKAYA, I., ATKIN, A., HORVATH, F., UNO, M. and BROOKS, V.B. Reversible movement dis-orders during cooling of n. dentatus. *Excerpta Medica Int. Congress Series*, **1969**, *193*: 241.
KOZLOVSKAYA, I., HORVATH, F., ATKIN, A. and BROOKS, V.B. Effect of dentate cooling on motor per-formance during afferent deprivation. *Physiologist*, **1970**a, *13*: 244.
KOZLOVSKAYA, I., UNO, M., ATKIN, A. and BROOKS, V.B. Performance of a step-tracking task by monkeys. *Comm. Behav. Biol.*, **1970**b, *5*: 153–156.
UNO, M., KOZLOVSKAYA, I., ATKIN, A. and BROOKS, V.B. Reversible movement disorders during cooling of the interposed nuclei. *Electroenceph. clin. Neurophysiol.*, **1971**, *31*: 298P.
WELT, C., ASCHOFF, J.C., KAMEDA, K. and BROOKS, V.B. Intracortical organization of cat's sen-sorimotor neurons. In D.P. PURPURA and M.D. YAHR (EDS.), *The neurophysiological basis of normal and abnormal motor activities*. Raven Press, New York, **1967**: 255–293.

Computer Analysis of the Clinical EEG [1]

A.O. BISHOP JR. AND W.P. WILSON

Department of Psychiatry, Duke University Medical Center and the VA Hospital, Durham, N. C. and the Department of Electrical Engineering, Clemson University, Clemson, S.C. (U.S.A.)

EEG records according to Cobb (1963) are read by determining (1) the frequency and amplitude of its rhythmic components, (2) the location and distribution of its rhythmic and transient components including bilateral symmetry, (3) the form of the rhythmic and transient components, and (4) their reactivity to the more commonly used activating techniques including eye-opening, hyperventilation, intermittent photic stimulation and sleep. The trained electroencephalographer obtains this information with ease, but as yet it has been impossible to find a method that will perform these tasks on a digital computer.

During the last two years (Bishop *et al.* 1969; Bishop *et al.* 1971), considerable effort has been expended in developing a computational method that promises to perform most of the tasks described by Cobb (1963). It is the purpose of this essay to summarize these efforts to date.

METHODS AND INSTRUMENTATION

Analytic techniques in on-line, real-time computer applications are selected according to (1) the information required and (2) the time consumed in the inherent mathematical manipulations. The information desired in the case of EEG is dependent on the frequency content of the wave form. The second consideration dictates a close study of frequency analysis techniques which require a minimum amount of computational time.

It has been shown that the frequency spectrums can be recovered from time-varying signals using a family of orthogonal square wave functions known as the Haar system (Hammond and Johnson 1962). Thus, retrieval of the frequency information content of the EEG is possible using this type of function. The applicability of this system is enhanced by a unique property which it possesses. Members of this system assume a single magnitude with either a positive or negative sign. Hence, a multiplication of the signal by any member of this system is reduced to a simple sign change. This most time-consuming mathematical operation, multiplication, is thereby reduced

[1] This work was supported in part by a contract with the National Air Pollution Control Administration, CPA-70-13.

References p. 129

to one of the most basic and fastest manipulations which can be performed on the digital computer, the addition of a number or its two's complement to other sums.

Additional work (Bishop 1969) has shown that the application of a similar system augmented by an ancillary time quadrature family of functions can be implemented in a series of digital filters. This type of filter provides a means of transforming the frequency and energy information content of the EEG signal into a quantitative statement about the signal. These filters unlike analog filters can be employed at very low frequencies with absolute gain and pass band stability and can be relied upon to produce accurate results in a fast computational mode as required by on-line, real-time analysis.

Briefly, this new family of functions and the ancillary time quadrature family of functions are defined by:

$$A(N, t) = \frac{1}{\sqrt{T}} \begin{cases} +2^{N/2} \text{ for } -aT \leq t \leq o \\ -2^{N/2} \text{ for } 0 \leq t \leq aT \\ 0 \text{ elsewhere} \end{cases}$$

and

$$B(N, t) = \frac{1}{\sqrt{T}} \begin{cases} 2^{N/2} \text{ for } -aT \leq t \leq -aT/2 \\ -2^{N/2} \text{ for } -aT/2 \leq t \leq aT/2 \\ 2^{N/2} \text{ for } aT/2 \leq t \leq aT \\ 0 \text{ elsewhere} \end{cases}$$

respectively, where $a = 2^{-N-1}$ and $N = 0, 1, 2$, *etc.* Fig. 1, *a* illustrates A(O, t), A(l, t), B(O, t) and B(l, t).

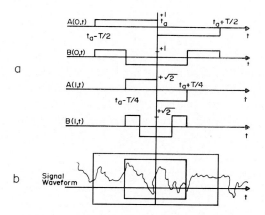

Fig. 1. *a*. Graphic illustration of *A* (o,t), *etc*. *b*. Action of filter on wave form at time t_a.

The magnitude of the Nth order complex coefficient, σ_N defined by these families for signal, f(t), is

$$\sigma_N = [A(N, t) f(t)]^2 + [B(N, t) f(t)]^2 \qquad \text{(Fig. 2)}$$

The transfer characteristic of this complex filter centered at 10 c/sec is illustrated in Fig. 3.

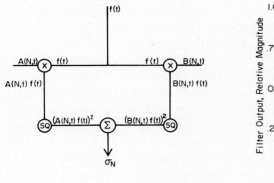
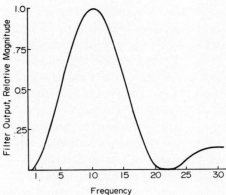

Fig. 2. Pictorial representation of Nth order complex coefficient.

Fig. 3. Transfer characteristics of filter at 10 c/sec.

Examine the case where the frequency band of interest is centered at 10 c/sec. The transfer function of the filter sets forth a required sampling interval of T = 0.092091 sec. This figure was obtained by computing the sampling interval for which the filter output is maximum at a center frequency of 10 c/sec. Pictorially, the action of this complex filter on the wave form to be analyzed at time t_a is shown above (Fig. 1, *b*).

As stated before, the multiplication of the signal, f(t), by the two functions A(N, t) and B(N, t) by the computer is accomplished by a sign change of the value of the signal from t_a to $t_a + T$ and $t_a — T/2$ to $t_a + T/2$, respectively, as these are the intervals over which A(N, t) and B(N, t) take on a non-zero value other than plus one.

The table below gives relative values of σ computed for a square, triangle and sine wave with a fundamental frequency of 10 c/sec as quantified by the filter centered at 10 c/sec.

	Max. value	Min. value	σ/T
Square wave form	1	−1	1
Triangular wave form	1	−1	.25
Sine wave form	1	−1	.404

Note that the measured values of σ/T represent the relative average squared values of these signals. For visual displays of the digital filter outputs, sine wave inputs have been used as reference. In clinical EEG analysis applications, an epoch of the resting–waking record is used to set a reference power level for each subject.

Transient analysis

The visual techniques used to analyze transients in EEG records can be described as perusing the record until some portion is spotted which does not fit the continuity of the record. This small portion is then isolated while checking the record before and after the anomaly. Once the decision is made that the isolated segment does in fact

References p. 129

qualify as a transient, attention is focused on the segment and an analysis of the transient begins. This analysis extracts significant information with regard to the transient activity such as amplitude, energy level, and frequency content.

The most difficult task assigned to the computer is the detection of anomalies. The method applied in the Fourier technique is the epoch analysis. Epoch analysis is defined as the analytical technique which is applied to successive non-overlapping epochs of records. The problem which arises when trying to implement this type of analysis while attempting to simulate the visual technique is that the human eye utilizes a method of analyzing continually varying lengths of record. Since the epoch analysis uses fixed intervals, transient activity which may appear arbitrarily in the epoch is subject to being completely masked by the redundant portion of the epoch. The approach taken in this new technique to simulate the visual scoring is to use successive overlapping epochs. After analyzing one epoch, less than 1% of the preceding epoch is moved out and new material amounting to less than 1% of the time interval under analysis is moved into the new epoch. A movie represents an example of the use of successive overlapping of pictures to provide motion. In this case, a perusal of two successive frames illustrates the fact that only a relatively small amount of information is added to or taken away from each successive picture. This technique is comparable to a moving window passing along the record and is referred to as the moving window technique. Fig. 4 illustrates the window moving along the time axis of a signal wave form.

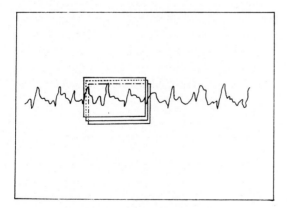

Fig. 4. Window moving along time axis of a signal.

As the window is moved along the record and passes in front of a transient, the analysis will be affected most when the window is centered on the transient. For this window position, a number is generated which describes the transient. The only time that a similar number will be generated is when a like transient appears in the window. In order to classify this transient more accurately, several windows of different widths are employed to view the transient and each in turn generates its own definitive number for the transient. Fig. 1, *b* illustrates the window enveloping a signal wave form for N = 0 and N = 1. As in the case of requiring an infinite number of coefficients to exactly describe a wave form using the Fourier technique, an infinite number of windows might be required here. However, due to the low resolution property of these windows, only a finite number is used to classify the few transients necessary for accurate sleep scoring. In fact, only 5 windows have been used thus far to achieve distinction between the 6 levels of sleep. Hence, 5 numbers are used to identify each type of transient.

Using this technique, information pertaining to the frequency of occurrence of similar transient activity can be extracted from the EEG record. If the response is evoked by using some activation procedure, the time between the stimulus and different portions of the response is measurable. No additional computations are required to obtain this datum as it is proportional to the time between an integer number of sampling intervals.

The computations required using the set of functions described can be performed fast enough to allow the implementation of the moving window technique. Hence, this technique closely parallels the electroencephalographer's visual technique and, as will be shown later in this essay, agrees with his analysis of the EEG record.

General pattern classification

The two distinct problems associated with pattern classification as defined by Ho and Agrawala (1968) are: (1) the Characterization Problem and (2) the Abstraction and Generalization Problem.

The Characterization Problem is confined to converting the wave form, the EEG, into a set of features which characterize the wave form. This problem is simply a transformation or mapping of the information content of the original wave form into a more easily definable set of features. The amount of information contained in this set of features is less than that contained in the original wave form. This is normally the reason for resorting to a pattern classification scheme since the original wave form contains too much information for accurate discernment. However, these features must retain sufficient information from the original wave form for classification of the wave form.

The Abstraction Problem is associated with defining a decision surface which will separate or classify the original wave form into proper categories using the set of features defined in the characterization problem. The Generalization Problem is the screening procedure which evaluates the goodness of the decision surface for classifying the original wave form.

There is no clear cut distinction between the Characterization problem and the Abstraction and Generalization Problem. It is clear that both processes are necessary, but not sufficient although it is generally conceded that the abstraction problem is the focal point of pattern classification.

The major portion of this essay has been devoted to the characterization problems since it is felt that this is the area of interest and the place where more work needs to be done, especially when the pattern classification is to be accomplished in real time.

A brief description of the abstraction technique which has been implemented will now be reviewed. Certain patterns of the feature set were noted in connection with

References p. 129

levels of sleep as well as with artifact and epileptic discharge. The dimensionality of the vector described by the features characterized using the digital filters is 6. A physical interpretation of these features correlated with the original wave form is 5 frequency and energy sensitive filters whose characteristic has been shown in Fig. 3 which have center frequencies of 1.25 c/sec (σ_0), 2.5 c/sec (σ_1), 5 c/sec (σ_2), 10 c/sec (σ_3) and 20 c/sec (σ_4). The sixth feature, Σ, is the summation of the filter outputs averaged over a specified time interval depending on the type of analysis. Sleep records dictate a longer interval, *i.e.* one second, whereas normal EEG records including hyperventilation and photic stimulation require shorter intervals as transient activity becomes more meaningful.

A plot of the decision surface which is currently being screened is shown in Fig. 5.

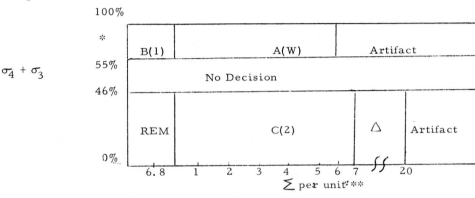

* % is based on ratio of $\sigma_4 + \sigma_3$ to $\sigma_0 + \sigma_1 + \sigma_2 + \sigma_3 + \sigma_4$.

** relative energy of a normalized section of A(W) record to the epoch being classified.

Fig. 5

D(3) and E(4) are distinguished by the number of 1-sec intervals in a 10-sec epoch in which the Δ decision is made.

Comparison of this decision surface with that illustrated by Larson and Walter (1970) shows a close resemblance in the shape of the surfaces and decisions made.

Epileptic discharges have been observed to structure a feature pattern which is high in σ_4 and σ_3 and is differentiated from artifact since this phenomenon shows an even distribution of the σ components. Both are high in the Σ component.

RESULTS

The information extraction considered desirable by Cobb (1963) has been developed as follows:

Form and repetition rate of rhythmic components
From the outset, it was recognized that a detailed analysis of the frequency spectrum

of the EEG was unnecessary. The electroencephalographer does not determine the frequency of every wave nor is he particularly interested in the variation of waves. He does, however, divide EEG frequencies into bands which have been designated by the familiar greek letters α, β, θ, Δ, and in sleep Σ. (This latter rhythm, it is recognized, is at the limit of the alpha range and is not solely defined by frequency.) The unique advantage of the analytic procedure described here is that it does determine the relative energy found in frequency bands much as the electroencephalographer might extract this information. More importantly, it performs the task in much the same way that he does by using a moving window, *i.e.*, he is constantly discarding old informa-

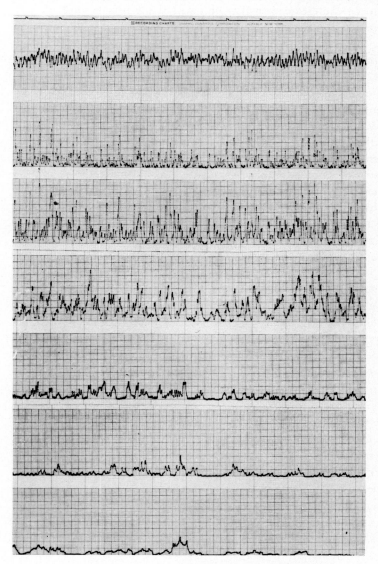

Fig. 6. Highly amplified outputs for σ, 1–6 of a normal EEG.

References p. 129

tion and adding new information as he scans a small section of the record. An example of this information extraction is provided in Fig. 6. It was determined, however, that information is not lost using this technique. Since the digital filters described are adaptable to power spectrum analysis we have compared the output of such a power spectrum with the Fourier power spectrum computed on a GASL analyzer. The similarity of the two analyses can be readily observed in Fig. 7 and corroborates the hypothesis that the digital filters extract information as does the Fourier power spectrum. The scaling of the computer output is amplified to demonstrate the considerable energy available in the signal in the bands of frequencies centering on 10 and 20 c/sec (σ_3 and σ_4). This picture is to be contrasted with that obtained in the fourth stage of sleep where the energy is centered in the 1.25, 2.5 and 5 bands (Fig. 8).

Form of transient components

Transient activity in the EEG falls into two categories. The first is due to noise arising primarily from non-cerebral sources. Examples are electrode pop artifact, ECG, muscle and movement artifact. The second are those events arising as a result of the increased discharge of aggregates of neurones firing in synchrony. These appear in the EEG as epileptic discharge. Visual analysis of these events at different cerebral levels indicates that the events recorded at the scalp are a synthesis of many events and may have a profile of energy in various frequency bands that would make them uniquely suited to analysis using a digital filtering technique. Such an approach would be more desirable than ones using the Fourier analysis with a short epoch, or a time-interval histogram. Both the time-interval histogram and the Fourier trigonometric analysis techniques are committed to an epoch type of analysis and due to their computational time requirements do not permit analysis of overlapping time intervals. In order to increase frequency resolution which is necessary for extracting transient information without introducing a narrow window, the analysis is applied to overlapping segments of the wave form. Thus, the transient is recognized as it is centered in the moving window and does not become masked in the background signal as in the usual (non-overlapping) epoch type of analysis. The rhythmic components of the signal are detected by nearly constant filter outputs whereas the transient components effect detectable output changes in the filter centered about the frequency band in which the spectrum of the particular transient resides. Hence, transients of several different bands of frequencies are made discernible rather than the recognition of only the high frequency variety. As it seemed likely that the complex filters described would recognize transient activity, an analysis of a number of transients were undertaken. Both noise and epileptic discharge were analyzed. The results of these analyses were encouraging and strongly suggested that artifacts would be readily distinguished from epileptic discharge because of definite characteristics exhibited by the complex filter outputs of these two distinct classes of input signals.

Location, distribution and bilateral symmetry of both rhythmic and transient components

Efforts to date using equipment available have been directed toward the analysis of 2

*G

TYPE IN DATA BY ROWS

```
:0,:1,:9,:63,:27,:53,
:0,:0,:7,:60,:33,:87,
:3,:1,:0,:60,:24,:55,
:6,:1,:9,:55,:28,:71,
:0,:0,:9,:55,:36,:51,
:0,:1,:6,:58,:36,:76,
:0,:0,:1,:54,:45,:35,
:0,:0,:3,:60,:37,:40,
:0,:0,:13,:60,:31,:85,
```

A(W)

```
=   0.01080   =   0.00466   =   0.06660   =   0.59140   =   0.32655
```

MIN=   0.03126 MAX=   0.68880 E. AVG.=   61.44450

```
=   1.00  =  0.03126  ***
=   2.00  =  0.08803  *******
=   3.00  =  0.17181  *************
=   4.00  =  0.27239  ********************
=   5.00  =  0.37283  ****************************
=   6.00  =  0.46712  ***********************************
=   7.00  =  0.54733  ******************************************
=   8.00  =  0.60898  **********************************************
=   9.00  =  0.65342  *************************************************
=  10.00  =  0.68005  **************************************************
=  11.00  =  0.68880  ***************************************************
=  12.00  =  0.67902  **************************************************
=  13.00  =  0.65087  *************************************************
=  14.00  =  0.60673  **********************************************
=  15.00  =  0.55118  ******************************************
=  16.00  =  0.49049  *************************************
=  17.00  =  0.43166  ******************************
=  18.00  =  0.38018  ***************************
=  19.00  =  0.33934  ************************
=  20.00  =  0.31073  **********************
=  21.00  =  0.29357  ********************
=  22.00  =  0.28603  ********************
=  23.00  =  0.28540  *******************
=  24.00  =  0.28862  *******************
=  25.00  =  0.29262  *******************
=  26.00  =  0.29438  *******************
=  27.00  =  0.29139  *******************
=  28.00  =  0.28204  *******************
=  29.00  =  0.26569  ******************
=  30.00  =  0.24285  *****************
=  31.00  =  0.21521  ***************
```

Fig. 7. Comparative power spectra using GASL analyzer and digital filter technique. GASL reads DC to 31 c/sec.

References p. 129

*G

TYPE IN DATA BY ROWS

```
:48,:22,:12,:12,:6,:185,
:55,:25,:19,:7,:3,:357,
:42,:25,:13,:13,:6,:323,
:15,:24,:24,:28,:19,:174,
:3,:19,:10,:58,:19,:65,
:61,:18,:12,:7,:3,:309,
:0,:0,:58,:24,:16,:233,
:0,:0,:60,:34,:6,:186,
:28,:0,:48,:19,:6,:246,
```

E (4)

```
=   0.34054  =   0.15169  =   0.26351  =   0.17510  ÷   0.06915
```

MIN=   0.05523 MAX=   0.36856 E. AVG.= 230.88900

```
=   1.00  =   0.35223  **********************************************
=   2.00  =   0.34881  **********************************************
=   3.00  =   0.32924  ********************************************
=   4.00  =   0.36856  ***************************************************
=   5.00  =   0.33013  *******************************************
=   6.00  =   0.33884  *******************************************
=   7.00  =   0.33814  *******************************************
=   8.00  =   0.27822  ************************************
=   9.00  =   0.23315  ****************************
=  10.00  =   0.19837  ************************
=  11.00  =   0.18966  ************************
=  12.00  =   0.19691  ************************
=  13.00  =   0.20316  ************************
=  14.00  =   0.19932  ************************
=  15.00  =   0.18096  ***********************
=  16.00  =   0.14964  *******************
=  17.00  =   0.12249  ***************
=  18.00  =   0.10167  **************
=  19.00  =   0.08125  ***********
=  20.00  =   0.07018  *********
=  21.00  =   0.06269  *********
=  22.00  =   0.06061  *********
=  23.00  =   0.06237  *********
=  24.00  =   0.06546  *********
=  25.00  =   0.07054  **********
=  26.00  =   0.07435  **********
=  27.00  =   0.07636  **********
=  28.00  =   0.07675  **********
=  29.00  =   0.07383  **********
=  30.00  =   0.06499  *********
=  31.00  =   0.05523  ********
```

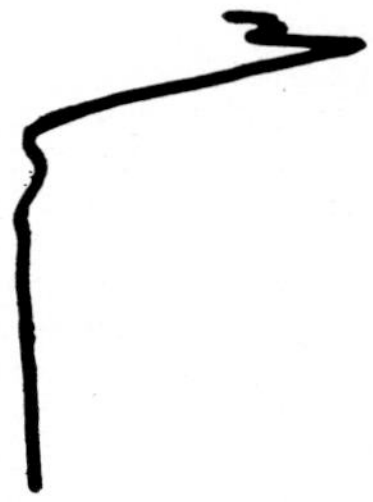

Fig. 8. Stage 4 sleep illustrating shift in energy using both GASL and digital filter techniques.

START

↓

Indicate electrode derivations to be auto-
matically programmed select classification
criteria for appropriate derivations in each
channel.

↓

Determine reference level from 10 to 30
seconds epoch of parieto-occipital derivation.

Introduce this into classification scheme as a
normal.

↓

If normalized epoch is not compatible for
indicated state of consciousness--then determine
appropriateness of gain.

↓

If appropriate--then proceed to determination
of appropriate classification of state of
consciousness--indicate--continuously assess
for change.

↓

Determine continually symmetry of homologous
areas and determine occurrence or lack of
occurrence of transients.

↓

If transients occur, determine characteristics
and classify if found in more than one channel--
determine phase relationships either in homologous areas or in contiguous areas.

↓

With appropriate screening runs--resting state
established.

↓

Technician--indicates beginning of hyperventilation.

↓

Computer--determines change if any occurs.

↓

Indicate--classify amount and nature of change.

↓

Technician--indicates end.

↓

Computer--determines persistance of change and
indicates.

↓

After appropriate resting period signal onset of
photic stimulation--determine nature of response
if any and classify if response occurs.

↓

Continue to screen all derivations for frequency
and amplitude of rhythmic components and occurrence
of transients--classify and indicate.

↓

STOP

Fig. 9. Flow chart of proposed analytic method for clinical EEG.

References p. 129

channels of information. With current computer capacity, it will be possible to analyze 4 channels. However, by multiplexing the inputs it will be further possible to do simultaneous analysis of homologous areas and extend the analytic capacity to 8 channels. With such capacity, the only limiting factor will be the fast accessible storage capacity necessary for implementation of pattern classification schemata.

The ability to perform multichannel analysis makes localization, lateralization and determination of bilateral synchrony quite readily possible. Here energy output in the various coefficients from homologous areas can be continuously compared with little additional computational requirement. These programs are to be developed.

Activating procedures

No effort has been made to develop specific techniques for these procedures as yet. Nevertheless, there should be no problem in the appropriate computational procedures for determining the pathological significance of the changes induced by hyperventilation and photic stimulation. The effects of sleep are considered necessary in basic EEG programs and results of sleep recognition will be reported in the near future.

SUMMARY AND CONCLUSIONS

Past and current efforts using Fourier power spectrum analysis for clinical EEG have been limited due to the considerable time necessary to perform the required arithmetical operations. It has been desirable then that a simple method be devised that can extract information rapidly and have adequate time for processing this information. The technique of digital filtering outlined here possesses this potential. As well it is uniquely adapted to pattern recognition programs that allow classification of transient events occurring in the EEG signal. The simplicity of the information extraction and pattern recognition process allows multichannel analysis on a modern minicomputer. Hardware modification with multiplexing will allow at least 8 channels of analysis to be performed simultaneously. This capacity allows judgements as to symmetry and localization of transients and effects of activating procedures to be made.

At the present stage of development the data extraction technique is clearly superior to Fourier techniques in terms of time requirements of computational capacity. The preliminary work performed on the pattern recognition techniques indicates that they have considerable probability of determining both the form and frequency of the rhythmic and transient components. As all other necessary analytic procedures will require only programming manipulations and equipment additions it is highly possible that the EEG can be analyzed for its information content within the next 3 years. It is unlikely that interpretation can be entrusted to a computer in the near future.

REFERENCES

BISHOP, A.O. *The development of an on-line, real-time digital computer technique for the analysis of electroencephalograms*. Ph.D. dissertation, Clemson University, **1969**: 17–20.

BISHOP, A.O., WILSON, W.P. and WILCOX, L.C. Use of the Haar function in automatic EEG analysis. *Electroenceph. clin. Neurophysiol.*, **1969**, *27*: 682.

BISHOP, A.O., SNELSIRE, R.W., WILCOX, L.C. and WILSON, W.P. The moving window approach to on-line, real-time waveform recognition. *Proc. 1970 San Diego Biomed. Symp.*, San Diego, Calif. **1971**.

COBB, W.A., The normal adult EEG. In H.D.N. HILL and G. PARR (EDS.), *Electroencephalography*. MacMillan, New York, **1963**: 232–249.

HAMMOND JR., J.L. and JOHNSON, R.S. A review of orthogonal square-wave functions and their application to linear networks. *J. Franklin Inst.*, **1962**, *273*: 211–225.

LARSON, L.E. and WALTER, D.O. On automatic methods of sleep staging by EEG spectra. *Electroenceph. clin. Neurophysiol.*, **1970**, *28*: 459–467.

HO, YU-CHI and AGRAWALA, A.K. On pattern classification algorithms. Introduction and survey. *TR No. 557, Div. of engr. and appl. physics*, Harvard University, Cambridge, Mass., **1968**.

Central and Peripheral Measures of Motivational States

JOHN R. KNOTT

Division of EEG and Neurophysiology, Department of Psychiatry, University of Iowa, College of Medicine, Iowa City, Iowa 52240 (U.S.A.)

The relationships between certain characteristics of the rhythmic components of the human and animal EEG and levels of cortical excitability were discussed by Herbert Jasper as early as 1936 (Jasper 1936). It was suggested that extreme levels of either negative or positive baseline shifts in the EEG might be related to depression of alpha activity, and that negative baseline shifts would be related to increased cortical excitability. In other observations demonstrated in the same report, Jasper related increased excitability to low voltage fast activity in the EEG. At least one causal variable for such increased excitability in the cat was shown to be a basic motivational, visceral drive state (need to micturate). Observations of this type did much to provide a foundation for developing conceptual bridges between brain activity and behavior.

In 1964, Walter *et al.* reported their discovery of the contingent negative variation (CNV), a slow (d.c.) potential shift which develops between the warning and imperative stimulus in a fixed foreperiod reaction time experiment. This very important finding certainly may be considered an extension of Jasper's original formulation of negative shifts related to increased excitability, since Walter *et al.* speculated that the CNV might serve as a mechanism for "priming" the cortex, and facilitating the processing of incoming information. McAdam (1969), indeed, has shown that certain components of evoked potentials have shorter latencies during the development of a CNV. Papakostopoulos *et al.* (1970) also reported data in keeping with this hypothesis, although some differences appear between McAdam's data and theirs.

Walter's initial impression was that the CNV, as an electrophysiological process, was related to "expectancy", as a psychological process. Other hypothetical constructs, or psychological variables, have also been implicated: "conation", "semantic value" and "attention", to name only a few.

Still another psychological variable which has been proposed as a correlate of the CNV is "motivation". Work in our laboratory (Irwin *et al.* 1966; Rebert *et al.* 1967; Knott and Irwin 1967; Chiorini 1969; McAdam *et al.* 1969; Rebert and Irwin 1969; Irwin and Rebert 1970) has led us to regard motivational states, both specific and nonspecific, as an important class of variables to be considered when seeking correlates of the CNV.

Our attention was particularly drawn to this when we used a differential paradigm (Irwin *et al.* 1966). When Tone$_1$ (the warning stimulus, S_1) was on the right, it indicated that the subject should press a key when the light (the imperative stimulus, S_2) followed, and there was a clearly definable CNV. However when $Tone_2$ (the warning) was on the left, it indicated that the subject was not to press the key when the light flashed, and there was a smaller CNV, although it was not absent. A related experiment utilized a differential warning signal, so that $Tone_1$ (left) indicated that the second stimulus would be a weak electrical shock, while $Tone_2$ (right) indicated that the second stimulus would be a noxious, unpleasant shock. Even though no manual response was required, CNVs developed between S_1 and the imperative stimulus. When the subjects were instructed to respond, the CNVs became larger. This experiment suggested to us that a drive state was being activated and that the CNV might be its directly observable correlate. Cant and Bickford (1967) have also implicated shock as a motivating variable, in an experiment in which the manual response, if appropriately timed, could serve to avoid the shock.

Chiorini (1969) was, at about the same time, carrying out observations on classical aversive conditioned responses (CRs) in the cat. He found that negative shifts developed in motor cortex, between the conditioned (CS) and the unconditioned stimulus (UCS), related to behavioral CRs (*i.e.* anticipatory leg flexion). Again, the evidence suggested motivational factors as being involved. Somewhat later, Irwin and Rebert (1970) and Rebert and Irwin (1969) studied appetitive CRs and subcortical slow potential shifts, using hunger as the motivating state. There was a relationship between the amount of food deprivation and the size of the voltage shift, reward being constant, which also pointed to motivational factors. Borda (1970), studying slow potential changes in monkey, did not find a simple relationship with drive. Indeed, he felt that "selective attention" might be the critical variable, and that it was the more direct correlate of food deprivation. However, if "selective attention" was the crucial variable, greater CNVs should occur than usually are seen in situations in which the subject must select a non-response as well as a response, since attention to the irrelevant stimulus is also required.

To some extent, the issue may be regarded, although not dismissed, as one of semantics. It is difficult to consider a state of attending without assuming a related state of motivation. Since in the basic CNV paradigm we encounter the development of a shift *before* the analog of the (or in some experiments, the actual) UCS, we have a model for a secondary drive state. The experiments involving shock can be interpreted as involving a "conditioned emotional reaction" or a "conditioned anxiety" state. Certainly attention and expectancy are involved, but McAdam *et al.* (1969) indicated that, statistically, only about 20% of the variance in their experiments could be attributed to such a variable, at least when reaction time and CNV were being related. A further analysis of their data suggested that the form of the CNV in time (comparing several intervals) resembled that of the psychologists' "goal gradient" and that the CNV reached a maximum when consummatory behavior would occur.

Taylor (1951) postulated "anxiety level" to be related to speed of learning of a classical aversive CR (eye closure). Using a scale drawn from items in the Minnesota Multiphasic Inventory by which to separate "anxious" and "non-anxious" normal subjects, she argued that the former would have an inherently high level of generalized drive and, when drive associated with a specific noxious stimulus (air puff) was added, acquisition of the aversive conditioned eye closure would be rapid, compared with a "non-anxious" group. This she clearly demonstrated.

Knott and Irwin (1967; 1968) argued that subjects with a "high anxiety" level, placed in the high shock (aversive) paradigm we had previously studied, should show larger CNVs than non-anxious subjects. However, this was not the case. In fact, while "low anxiety" subjects and "high anxiety" subjects did not differ in a paradigm using low stress (*i.e.*, in which the imperative stimulus was a tone), the differences we had predicted were reversed under stress. Since we utilized the differential paradigm, the failure of our prediction was rather dramatic. With Warning$_1$: High Intensity shock signifying *no response* to shock (*i.e.*, no key press after shock) and Warning$_2$: High Intensity Shock signifying *response* to shock, the low anxiety subjects had larger CNVs in the response condition. The anxious subjects on the other hand, showed equally large CNVs in *both* conditions (Fig. 1).

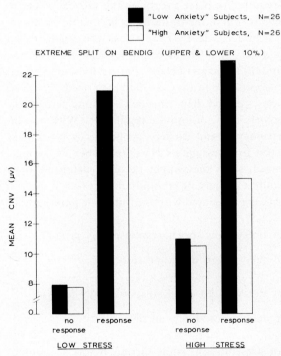

Fig. 1. CNVs under "low" and "high" stress, for "low anxiety" and "high anxiety" subjects, defined as low and high 10% scores on the Bendig Scale. (Based on data of Knott and Irwin 1968.)

In addition to measuring CNVs, galvanic skin responses (GSRs) were also recorded. Plotting them in terms of *anticipatory* responses, that is in terms of percent CRs, no relationship could be demonstrated between CNV and GSR. While the high anxiety and low anxiety subjects were discriminated by their CNV behavior, they were not discriminated by their GSR behavior. To this degree, then, that peripheral autonomic measure failed to relate to the measure of motivational state. The central measure did discriminate.

References pp. 136–137

This was interpreted to be due to the fact that high anxiety subjects operate nearer to their maximum negative cortical level in all situations and that when they are stressed (and develop a diffuse conditioned emotional response) the shift goes to or nearly to the maximum. When the "response" condition is added, no further shift can be developed.

It has recently been possible to explore this problem from another angle of attack[1]. Instead of polarizing subjects into high anxiety *vs.* low anxiety as had been done before, an attempt was made to polarize them in terms of "perceptual style" (Witkin *et al.* 1962). Witkin has developed a scale of "field dependency" which categorizes subjects on the degree to which they respond to parts of the perceptual field on the basis of, or independently of, other parts of the field. The so-called "Rod and Frame Test" is used for this classification. Using a luminous frame which can be positioned at an angle to true horizontal, a luminous rod is placed within it, and positioned away from the true vertical. The subject and equipment is in total darkness, except for the luminous outline of rod and frame. The subject is required to place the rod in the vertical position. Subjects who are so influenced by the position of the frame as to be unable to do so, within a few degrees, are regarded as "field dependent" (FD). Those who can disregard the frame and rotate the rod to within a very small error of the vertical, are regarded as "field independent" (FI). Witkin and his associates believe that persons so grouped "resembled one another in particular aspects of *how* they satisfied their needs, resolved their conflicts, handled their aggressions, formed their attitudes". Among personality attributes believed to cluster together were those of impulse regulation (Witkin *et al.* 1962, p.8). Some equation of field dependency and anxiety proneness is postulated (*ibid.*, p.168). Thus, it seemed of interest to investigate CNVs, and other physiological variables, in groups so dichotomized, since they might be more definitive than those chosen on a simple scale of manifest anxiety or emotionality.

The subjects (N = 34; 17 FD, 17 FI) were presented with the following paradigm:

Day 1   High frequency tone–(3 sec delay)–low shock–response (key press)

          Low frequency tone–(3 sec delay)–high shock–no response

Day 2   High frequency tone–(3 sec delay)–high shock–response (key press)

          Low frequency tone–(3 sec delay)–low shock–no response

Group A received the above order of presentation, while Group B was a counter-balanced group, receiving the "Day" schedule in reverse order. In addition to measure of CNV, GSP (from left middle finger and forearm) and heart rate, were measured.

The FI and FD groups were compared on CNV scores (Fig. 2). The FI group show-

[1] The following experimental data were obtained during 1969–70, when I was a Visiting Professor in the Department of Psychiatry and Biobehavioral Sciences, and the Department of Neurology, Louisiana State University School of Medicine, New Orleans. Drs. Sanford Cohen, William van Veen and Lyle Miller were co-investigators. Mr. Jon Peters, Research Assistant, served as an active collaborator. The work was supported in part by Grant No. MH-18368-01, Mental Health Small Grants Committee, N.I.M.H.

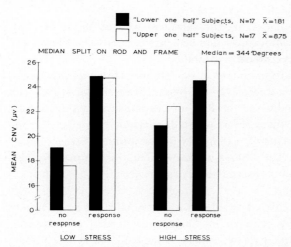

Fig. 2. Mean values of CNV for "low stress", no response and response conditions, and "high stress", no response and response conditions, for "field independent" (FI, lower half) and "field dependent" (FD, upper half) Rod and Frame Groups. The FI response *vs.* non-response difference, in both low and high stress conditions, is significant. The FD group did not show significant differences between non-response and response conditions in either low or high stress.

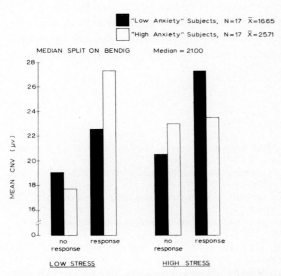

Fig. 3. Mean values of CNV for "low stress" no response and response conditions, and "high stress" no response and response conditions, for "low anxiety" (lower half) and "high anxiety" (upper half) (Bendig grouping).

ed a significant increase in CNV, in response as compared to non-response, under low stress ($P<0.02$) and stress ($P<0.05$). The FD group, on the other hand, did not show significantly greater CNVs in response conditions under either low or high Stress ($P > 0.05$ for both). The failure to achieve significance in the FD group appears to be due to excessive variances. Seven FD subjects had lower CNVs in stress–response than stress–non-response. Six had larger CNVs in the low stress–non-response condition.

References pp. 136–137

Although apparent differences occur in GSP, the variances were so large, and the means so small, that no statistical significance could be demonstrated. The FI and FD subjects were not different with respect to cardiac lability.

The data were then re-sorted, utilizing "anxiety" or "emotionality", as previously defined by Knott and Irwin (1968) on the basis of the Bendig Scale (Bendig 1962). No relationship was found between Bendig and the Rod and Frame test classification of the subjects. The CNV data resolved themselves essentially as would be predicted from the earlier work (Fig. 3). The "high anxiety", response $vs.$ non-response difference under stress was not significant ($P > 0.05$). The GSP responses were not discriminatory. The cardiac rate data were similarly without discriminatory function.

The weight of the evidence provided by these observations supports the conclusion that a relationship exists between CNV behavior and "anxiety proneness" in conditions of stress. The degree to which cognitive style (as defined by the Rod and Frame Test to determine field dependence and field independence) is related to CNV measures appears more complex. Certainly, as far as CNV measures are involved, field dependence is not related to anxiety-proneness. Hence, these two means of categorizing subjects are not equivalent. Since the evidence from Taylor's much earlier work indicates that there is reason to believe that level of anxiety-proneness is related to the psychological variable of motivation, a relationship between CNV and motivational state also seems to be probable. However, under the conditions of these experimental designs, peripheral measures such as skin potential and cardiac lability have no apparent relationship to such variables associated with CNV.

REFERENCES

BENDIG, A.W. The Pittsburgh scales of social extroversion-introversion and emotionality. *J. Psychol.*, **1962**. *53*: 199–209.

BORDA, R.P. The effect of altered drive states on the contingent negative variation (CNV) in rhesus monkeys. *Electroenceph. clin. Neurophysiol.*, **1970**, *29*: 173–180.

CANT, B.R. and BICKFORD, R.G. The effect of motivation on the contingent negative variation (CNV). *Electroenceph. clin. Neurophysiol.*, **1967**, *23*: 594.

CHIORINI, J.R. Slow potential changes from cat cortex and classical aversive conditioning. *Electroenceph. clin. Neurophysiol.*, **1969**, *26*: 399–405.

HEIN, P.L., COHEN, S.I. and SHMAVONIAN, B.M. Perceptual mode and Pavlovian typology. In J. WORTIS (Ed.), *Recent advances in biological psychiatry, Vol. 7*. Plenum Press, New York, **1964**: 71–78.

HILLYARD, S.A. Relationships between the contingent negative variation (CNV) and reaction time. *Physiol. & Behav.*, **1969**, *4*: 351–357.

IRWIN, D.A. and REBERT, C.S. Slow potential changes in cat brain during classical appetitive conditioning of jaw movements using two levels of reward. *Electroenceph. clin. Neurophysiol.*, **1970**, *28*: 119–126.

IRWIN, D.A., KNOTT, J.R., McADAM, D.W. and REBERT, C.S. Motivational determinants of the "contingent negative variation". *Electroenceph. clin. Neurophysiol.*, **1966**, *21*: 538–543.

JASPER, H.H. Cortical excitatory state and synchronism in the control of bioelectric autonomous rhythms. *Cold Spring Harbor Symposia on Quantitative Biology*, **1936**, *4*: 320–338.

KNOTT, J.R. and IRWIN, D.A. Anxiety, stress and the contingent negative variation. *Electroenceph. clin. Neurophysiol.*, **1967**, *22*: 188.

KNOTT, J.R. and IRWIN, D.A. Anxiety, stress and the contingent negative variation. *Electroenceph. clin. Neurophysiol.*, **1968**, *24*: 286–287.

Low, M.D. and McSherry, J.W. Further observations of psychological factors involved in CNV genesis. *Electroenceph. clin. Neurophysiol.*, **1968**, *25*: 203–207.

McAdam, D.W. Increases in CNS excitability during negative cortical slow potentials in man. *Electroenceph. clin. Neurophysiol.*, **1969**, *26*: 216–219.

McAdam, D.W., Knott, J.R. and Rebert, C.S. Cortical slow potential changes in man related to interstimulus interval and to pre-trial prediction of interstimulus interval. *Psychophysiology*, **1969**, *5*: 349–358.

Papakostopoulos, D., Walter, W. G. and Crow, H.J. The effect of stimulus context on evoked responses in human frontal cortex. *Electroenceph. clin. Neurophysiol.*, **1970**, *29*: 327–328.

Rebert, C.S. and Irwin, D.A. Slow potential changes in cat brain during classical appetitive and aversive conditioning of jaw movement. *Electroenceph. clin. Neurophysiol.*, **1969**, *27*: 152–161.

Rebert, C.S., McAdam, D.W., Knott, J.R. and Irwin, D.A. Slow potential change in human brain related to level of motivation. *J. comp. physiol. Psychol.*, **1967**, *63*: 20–23.

Taylor, J.A. The relationship of anxiety to the conditioned eyelid response. *J. exp. Psychol.*, **1951**, *41*: 81–92.

Walter, W.G., Cooper, R., Aldridge, V.J., McCallum, W.C. and Winter, A.L. Contingent negative variation: An electric sign of sensori-motor association and expectancy in the human brain. *Nature (Lond.)*, **1964**, *203*: 380–384.

Witkin, H.A., Dyk, R.B., Faterson, H.F., Goodenough, D.R. and Karp, S.A. *Psychological differentiation*. John Wiley, New York, **1962**.

Sélectivité Ionique et Réponses Electriques des Membranes Lipidiques Artificielles Excitables

A. M. MONNIER

Laboratoire de Physiologie Générale, Faculté des Sciences de Paris, 9, Quai St.-Bernard, Paris, 9e (France)

Ce mémoire porte sur les membranes "artificielles", c'est-à-dire sur un sujet qui diffère de tous ceux que ce recueil présente en affectueux hommage à Herbert Jasper. Cependant j'ai bonne excuse, car voici 35 ans nous avons sacrifié ensemble à l'artificialité. Nous avons alors formé avec des nerfs d'Invertébrés marins, la première synapse artificielle. C'était dans le petit laboratoire électroencéphalographique que H. H. Jasper avait aménagé dans une institution hospitalière de Providence, Rhode Island, l'Emma Pendleton Bradley Home, agréablement située au bord d'une baie tranquille, propice à l'immersion d'un vivier improvisé.

En 1936 Danielli a proposé une structure schématique de la membrane cellulaire, généralement admise aujourd'hui. Cette membrane serait constituée de deux feuillets monomoléculaires de phosphoaminolipides, accolés l'un à l'autre par leurs chaines lipidiques. *A priori*, selon la physique des phénomènes de surface, une telle membrane est instable si les feuillets sont à l'état liquide. Aussi Danielli supposait l'existence d'une couche protéique recouvrant les faces ioniques des deux feuillets de la membrane. Cette double couche protéique servirait en quelque sorte de squelette et donnerait la stabilité de forme à la membrane et, en outre, serait évidemment essentielle à la diversité de toutes les fonctions de celle-ci. En 1962, Mueller *et al.* réussirent à former entre deux solutions aqueuses des membranes stables, formées uniquement de deux feuillets lipidiques monomoléculaires. De nombreux auteurs ont étudié celles-ci. Leurs propriétés dépendent largement de leur constitution et notamment des additifs variés qu'il est nécessaire d'y inclure. Leur épaisseur infime (100 Å environ) est précisément de l'ordre de celle des membranes cellulaires. Malgré cela elles sont très peu conductrices. Leur structure est vraisemblablement très compacte, proche de l'état solide, ce qui expliquerait leur stabilité. La perméabilité de ces membranes ne devient notable qu'à la suite d'inclusion préalable de molécules particulières (antibiotiques macrocycliques) de structure annulaire, susceptible de sertir, en quelque sorte, un cation tel que K^+ et de le rendre liposoluble. L'inclusion d'un facteur protéique, de nature encore indéterminée, peut rendre la membrane électriquement excitable. Elle présente alors, en effet, sous l'action d'un champ électrique assez fort, des variations rythmées de conductance (Mueller et Rudin 1967). Des revues récentes (Bangham

1968; Mueller et Rudin 1968a, b) exposent l'ensemble des propriétés des couches bimoléculaires.

Les recherches de notre laboratoire depuis 1956 suivent une direction semblable, quoique différente. Nous avons supposé que la sélectivité ionique et l'excitabilité électrique des membranes cellulaires pourraient ne pas dépendre essentiellement d'une couche bimoléculaire, c'est-à-dire d'un "état de surface" particulier, mais plutôt des propriétés de la membrane considérée dans sa masse. Nous avons donc cherché à obtenir des membranes lipidiques artificielles ayant les caractères suivants: (1) solidité suffisante, pour séparer deux solutions aqueuses distinctes, (2) hydratation modérée, (3) présence de charges anioniques. Ces deux dernières conditions étant nécessaires à la perméabilité de la membrane aux cations.

Nous avons d'abord fait appel à des esters phosphoriques d'alcools gras et à du monooléate de glycérol, additionné d'un peu d'acide gras. Ces corps, en présence d'eau forment des gels peu hydratés, qui peuvent être mis sous forme de membranes.

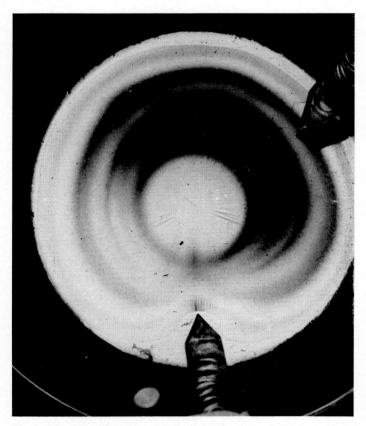

Fig. 1. Membrane formée par étalement d'une goutte d'huile de lin à la surface d'une solution de MnO_4K, 4 g/l et transférée à la surface d'une solution saline. Une électrode Ag-AgCl-KCl, située au bas de l'image, plonge dans cette dernière solution. Une électrode identique (en haut et à droite), est en contact avec une goutte de solution saline déposée à la surface de la membrane. Deux phases aqueuses distinctes reliées chacune à une électrode, sont ainsi séparées par la membrane.

Mais les membranes artificielles qui nous ont paru les plus intéressantes sont les suivantes, dont le présent article donne une revue générale de leurs propriétés principales.

LES MEMBRANES ARTIFICIELLES FORMEES A PARTIR DE LIPIDES NON SATURES

Nous avons songé à utiliser un triglycéride constitué par des acides gras non saturés, tels que l'huile de lin. En effet cette huile, employée depuis un temps immémorial par les peintres, étalée au pinceau sur un support, y forme peu à peu une membrane solide. Le "séchage" de l'huile de lin est, en réalité, une polymérisation oxydative sous l'effet de l'air, qui transforme la couche d'huile en un réseau tridimensionnel superficiel, où sont fixés des groupes peroxydes, aldéhydes, alcools et acides. *A priori*, une telle membrane paraissait intéressante à étudier, mais il est très difficile de la détacher de son support. Nous avons usé d'un procédé tout différent. Une goutte d'huile de lin, déposée à la surface d'une solution oxydante (MnO_4K à 1 g/l), s'y étale très rapidement et prend l'aspect d'une membrane circulaire de 10 à 15 cm de diamètre sur laquelle apparaissent de belles franges d'interférences, ce qui permet d'estimer sa très faible épaisseur, laquelle peut être inférieure à 1μ (Fig. 1) (Monnier et Monnier 1964). Au bout de quelques heures (ce temps dépend notamment de la température) la membrane est suffisamment solide pour qu'on puisse aspirer la solution oxydante et remplacer celle-ci par une solution saline quelconque. En outre, la membrane peut supporter, sans se rompre, une goutte d'une autre solution. Nous avons ainsi une membrane séparant deux phases aqueuses distinctes. Dans chacune de celle-ci on insère une électrode Ag-AgCl-KCl. Ces électrodes permettent la mesure précise des différences de potentiel de part et d'autre de la membrane et sont impolarisables par le courant. Dès nos premiers essais, de multiples analogies apparurent (Monnier *et al.* 1965a, b).

1. Si la membrane sépare deux solutions d'un même chlorure alcalin, mais de concentrations C_1 et C_2 différentes, on observe une différence de potentiel E_{mv} très voisine de celle donnée par la formule classique:

$$E_{mv} = 58,5 \log_{10} \frac{C_1}{C_2}$$

la solution la plus diluée étant positive. Ceci indique une sélectivité exclusive à l'endroit des cations et par conséquent, révèle l'existence de charges anioniques fixes au sein de la membrane. Ces charges résultent évidemment de la polymérisation oxydative préalable qui a formé cette dernière.

2. Si la membrane sépare des solutions de chlorure de cations différents, mais de même concentration, on observe une différence de potentiel notable, comme celle qu'on observe lorsqu'on étudie, dans les mêmes conditions, les membranes échangeuses de cations, de fabrication industrielle. Sollner (1949) a dénommé "potentiel bi-ionique" cette différence de potentiel, et l'attribue à ce que les "nombres de transport" des deux cations au sein de la membrane sont inégaux. Quand de part et d'autre de la membrane d'huile de lin, sont appliquées une solution de KCl et une solution de NaCl, à la même concentration, cette dernière solution est positive (E = 55 mV en moyenne).

Le rapport des nombres de transport à travers la membrane serait donné par la formule de Sollner:

$$\log_{10} \frac{T_K}{T_{Na}} = \frac{E_{mv}}{58,5} \text{ d'où } \frac{T_K}{T_{Na}} = 8,7 \text{ en moyenne ce qui montre que la membrane,}$$

comme celle des fibres nerveuses au repos, est beaucoup plus perméable aux ions K^+ qu'aux ions Na^+. Autrement dit la membrane manifeste une sélectivité intercationique.

a. *Perméabilité spécifique vis à-vis des divers cations alcalins* (Goudeau 1967a). Celle-ci est estimée, de manière relative, d'après le potentiel bi-ionique observé lorsqu'un côté de la membrane est en contact avec une solution de chlorure du cation considéré, l'autre étant baigné par une solution de LiCl a la même concentration (0,1 M). Les membranes sont formées par une goutte d'un mélange à parts égales, d'huile de lin et d'huile d'oïticica, étalée sur une solution de MnO4K. Ces membranes donnent des potentiels bi-ioniques plus faibles que celles formées d'huile de lin pure, mais plus réguliers. Dans tous les cas, le côté Li^+ de la membrane s'est montré positif. Donc, pour ce cation, la membrane présente la plus faible perméabilité. Les potentiels bi-ioniques E_{mv}, et les rapports des nombres de transport, par rapport à Li^+, se classent selon la séquence suivante:

	Na^+	NH_4^+	K^+	Rb^+	Cs^+
$E_{mv} =$	14	43	55	62	69
$\dfrac{T_{m^+}}{T_{Li^+}} =$	1,7	5,5	8,8	11,8	15,3

Ainsi les cations de poids atomique élevé passent plus aisément à travers la membrane. Ce sont donc les cations les plus petits, c'est-à-dire les plus volumineux parce que les plus hydratés, qui franchissent la membrane le plus difficilement (Fig. 2).

Si on ajuste le pH des solutions en contact avec la membrane, au moyen d'une faible addition de solution tampon, on constate que ce facteur a une grande influence sur la conductance de la membrane. La figure 3 montre que la conductance, calculée d'après la caractéristique courant-tension, augmente tout au long de la gamme des pH étudiés (pH 2,50 à 8,85). Mais l'augmentation de conductance n'est sensible qu'à partir de pH 4,75. Au pH 8,85, la membrane peut être dix fois plus conductrice qu'au pH 4,75. Mais la membrane présente alors un gonflement perceptible qui annonce sa désintégration. Aux pH supérieurs à 10 le gonflement s'accuse beaucoup et la membrane s'effrite rapidement. La sélectivité vis-à-vis des cations alcalins présente un maximum entre pH 4 et pH 6. La sélectivité intercationique (estimée d'après la mesure des potentiels bi-ioniques) atteint son maximum entre les mêmes pH. On peut en déduire que les sélectivités dépendent de la présence d'une certaine quantité d'eau dans la membrane. On peut penser que cette hydratation est modérée, mais suffisante pour provoquer l'ionisation d'une partie des groupes acides fixés à la membrane.

b. *Perméabilité spécifique vis-à-vis des cations organiques monovalents* (Goudeau, 1967b). Comme ci-dessus une face de la membrane est en contact avec le chlorure du cation envisagé, l'autre face avec du ClLi, à la même concentration. Cette dernière

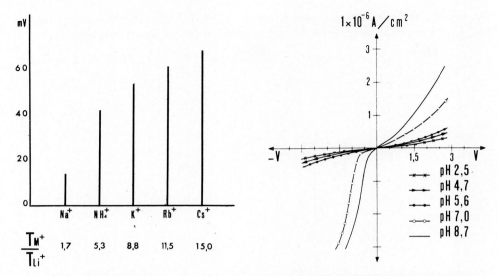

Fig. 2. Potentiels bi-ioniques par rapport au Li$^+$ dus à divers cations inorganiques monovalents. La membrane sépare, dans chaque cas, une solution de chlorure du cation considéré et une solution du LiCl à la même concentration. Ces potentiels montrent que la perméabilité relative de la membrane, par rapport au Li$^+$, s'élève avec la masse atomique du cation.

Fig. 3. Caractéristique courant-voltage d'une membrane formée d'un mélange à part égale d'huile de lin et d'huile d'oïticica. Cette caractéristique devient non linéaire dès que le voltage s'élève.

On notera l'influence du pH. Pour le pH 8,7, seule l'allure de la courbe est donnée, car la caractéristique se modifie alors rapidement pendant les mesures.

face est toujours positive pour tous les cations organiques étudiés. Le nombre de transport (calculé selon la formule de Sollner) et par conséquent la perméabilité de la membrane, sont donc, pour ces cations, toujours plus élevés que pour le Li$^+$. Le rapport entre le nombre de transport T_M^+ du cation considéré, et celui T_{Li}^+ du lithium, augmente avec le nombre des radicaux liés à l'azote du cation organique.

	NH_4^+	Diméthyl NH_2^+	Triméthyl NH^+	Tétraméthyl N^+
$\dfrac{T_M^+}{T_{Li}^+} =$	3,60	10,5	12,0	14,1

Il croit de même avec la masse de ces radicaux.

	NH_4^+	Ethyl NH_3^+	Triéthyl NH^+	Tétraéthyl N^+
$\dfrac{T_M^+}{T_{Li}^+} =$	3,60	10,5	35,5	39,8

Le rapport entre les nombres de transport s'élève beaucoup avec la longueur des radicaux attachés à l'azote.

	NH_4^+	Tétraméthyl N^+	Tétraéthyl N^+	Tétrabutyl N^+
$\dfrac{T_M^+}{T_{Li}^+} =$	3,55	10,5	81,0	1180,0

De même, certaines drogues cationiques se caractérisent aussi par des potentiels bi-ioniques et donc des nombres de transport remarquablement élevés (Fig. 4).

	Hexaméthonium$^+$	Acétylcholine$^+$	Guanidine$^+$	Ephédrine$^+$
$\dfrac{T_{M^+}}{T_{Li^+}} =$	1,60	44	113	224

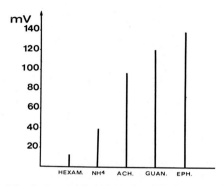

Fig. 4. Potentiels bi-ioniques par rapport au Li$^+$ dûs à quelques drogues cationiques monovalentes: héxaméthonium, ammoniaque, acétylcholine, guanidine, éphédrine. La perméabilité relative de la membrane, par rapport au Li$^+$, est considérable pour celles-ci.

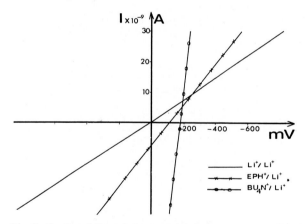

Fig. 5. Partie médiane de la caractéristique courant-tension d'une membrane d'huile de lin, dont une face est constamment en contact avec une solution de LiCl 0,1 M et l'autre face, en contact successivement avec des chlorures de Li$^+$, éphédrine$^+$, tétrabutylammonium$^+$ 0,1 M. Lorsque les cations de part et d'autre de la membrane sont différents, le potentiel pour la valeur 0 du courant est le potentiel bi-ionique (la face Li$^+$ étant toujours positive). La pente de la caractéristique, c'est-à-dire la conductance, augmente du fait de la présence d'un cation organique volumineux d'un côté de la membrane.

Ces cations organiques mettent en évidence un phénomène très curieux. Sur la même région de la membrane on applique d'abord des deux côtés une solution de LiCl. Puis, on remplace d'un seul côté cette solution par une solution contenant le cation organique à la même concentration; on constate que la conductance de cette region augmente. Elle double avec l'éphédrine et augmente près de 20 fois avec le tétra-butylammonium (Fig. 5). Le contact d'un gros cation organique d'un seul côté de la membrane peut donc modifier la structure de celle-ci. Il semble que les cations organiques chassent les cations alcalins de la membrane. Le courant à travers la membrane serait alors exclusivement porté par les cations organiques. Dans ce cas, la formule de Sollner qui exprime le potentiel bi-ionique est encore adéquate si on explicite les nombres de transport.

$$E_{mv} = 58,5 \log_{10} \frac{T_1}{T_2} = 58,5 \log_{10} \frac{C_1 U_1}{C_2 U_2}$$

U_1 et U_2, C_1 et C_2 étant respectivement les mobilités et les concentrations des cations organique et inorganique dans la membrane. Comme ci-dessus, les phases aqueuses au contact de la membrane contiennent, l'une les cations organiques, et l'autre les cations Li^+, à la même concentration. Si dans la membrane, la concentration C_2 des cations Li^+ est très faible par rapport à celle C_1 des cations organiques, c'est-à-dire si l'affinité de la membrane pour ces derniers est très forte ,le potentiel bi-ionique est élevé. Mais, d'autre part la conductance peut être très grande si les gros cations organiques possèdent une mobilité U_1 élevée dans la membrane. Une grande mobilité de ces cations peut, en effet, être envisagée car les contacts entre les radicaux alkyls attachés à l'azote et le réticulum lipidique de la membrane ne sont l'objet que de faibles forces de Van der Waals (Fig. 19).

Des résultats récents, dont l'analogie pharmacodynamique est évidente, montrent d'une manière encore plus frappante, l'action des cations organiques monovalents sur le potentiel bi-ionique et sur la conductance des membranes. On part d'une membrane séparant deux solutions identiques Li^+–Li^+. On ajoute d'une côté un colorant à très faible concentration, par exemple du chlorure de violet de méthyle à 10_{-4} M. En quelques minutes un potentiel bi-ionique de près de 300 mV s'établit (le côté contenant du Li^+ pur étant positif). La résistance, de 32 mégΩ au départ, tombe à 2,5 mégΩ environ Ce résultat s'interprète comme ci-dessus par l'effet d'un échange quasi total du Li^+ en faveur du cation violet de méthyle lequel, d'autre part, paraît avoir une grande mobilité au sein de la membrane (Fig. 6). Nous verrons plus loin qu'il s'agit là d'un véritable échange ionique entre les ions H des groupes acides fixés à la membrane et les cations organiques.

c. *Réduction de la perméabilité spécifique sous l'effet des cations inorganiques divalents* (Goudeau 1968). Si on place une solution contenant un peu de Ca^{++} au contact de la membrane, la résistance de la membrane s'élève beaucoup. Il semble donc que les cations Ca^{++} sont fortement liés aux charges anioniques fixées à la membrane, ce qui réduit évidemment leur mobilité (Fig. 7).

d. *Réduction de la perméabilité par de faibles traces de cations organiques divalents.* Dans ce cas les effects observés sont à l'opposé de ceux obtenus avec les cations monovalents. Si d'un côté d'une membrane entourée comme ci-dessus de solutions de LiCl 0,1 M, on ajoute une trace d'un cation organique divalent (par exemple, du chlorure de D-tubocurarine 10^{-5} M), les effets sont tout différents. Le potentiel bi-ionique n'excède guère 20 mV, mais, au bout de quelques heures, la résistance de la membrane augmente beaucoup; elle passe par exemple de 10 à 62 mégΩ. Dans ce cas encore, les cations organiques divalents paraissent envahir la membrane par suite d'un échange ionique aux dépens des groupes acides fixes. Mais, en raison de leurs doubles charges, les attractions électrostatiques les rendent peu mobiles d'où augmentation de la résistance de la membrane (Fig. 8).

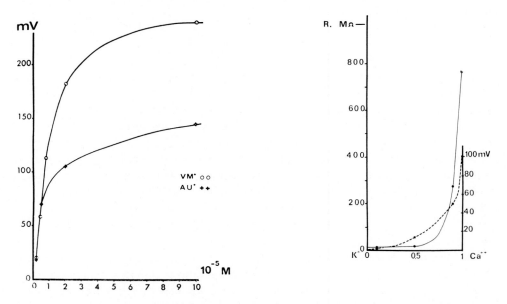

Fig. 6. Membrane d'huile de lin et d'huile d'oïticica séparant deux solutions initialement identiques du LiCl. De traces de cations organiques monovalents: violet de méthyl (VM⁺), auramine (Au⁺), sont ajoutés d'un côté de la membrane. On constate alors une différence de potentiel considérable entre les deux faces de la membrane, ce qui indique que ces cations organiques envahissent la membrane et y possèdent une grande mobilité. L'analogie pharmacodynamique est évidente.

Fig. 7. Membrane d'huile de lin dont une face est en contact avec KCl 0,1 M et l'autre avec un mélange de KCl et de CaCl₂ en proportion variable, mais à la même concentration totale équivalente. On voit qu'au fur et à mesure que la proportion de Ca⁺⁺ augmente, le potentiel bi-ionique (trait discontinu) se manifeste et la résistance de la membrane (trait plein) augmente considérablement. La face contenant du Ca⁺⁺ est toujours positive.

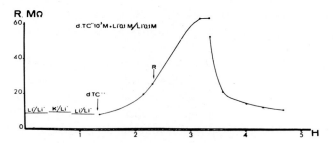

Fig. 8. Sous l'effet d'une trace d'un cation organique divalent d'un côté de la membrane (d-Tubocurarine), la résistance ⁽ᴿ⁾ de la membrane augmente considérablement.

En conclusion, ces divers effets si marqués, de traces de cations organiques sur les propriétés de la membrane évoquent, de manière frappante, les actions si importantes qu'exercent sur les fibres nerveuses, à très faibles doses, les agents pharmacodynamiques.

e. *Excitabilité électrique* (Monnier *et al.* 1965a, b; Reynier-Rebuffel 1968). Lorsque un faible courant établit une différence de potentiel de 100–200 mV (c'est-à-dire un champ électrique assez faible de quelques centaines de V/cm) de part et d'autre de la membrane, on observe une véritable "réponse" à l'excitation électrique (Fig. 9). La membrane présente alors des accroissements transitoires et répétés de *conductance* (Fig. 10). Le rythme de ces réponses croît avec la différence de potentiel, comme pour la membrane nerveuse. Comme pour celle-ci la relation rythme-voltage est linéaire sur une large étendue (Fig. 11). L'allure des réponses toutefois évoque plutôt celle de l'électrocardiogramme élémentaire (Fig. 12), analogue d'ailleurs à l'allure des "réponses" obtenues par Mueller et Rudin (1967, 1968b) sur des membranes bimoléculai

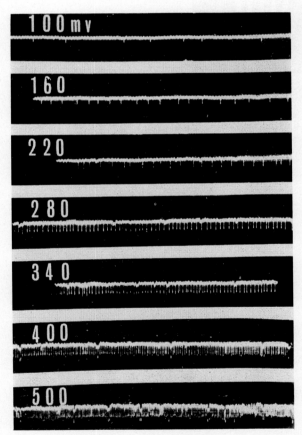

Fig. 9. Réponse rythmique d'une membrane d'huile de lin insérée entre deux solutions de KCl 0,1 M, sous des courants d'intensité croissante. Les chiffres indiquent la tension appliquée à la membrane dans chaque cas. Ces réponses sont des accroissements temporaires de conductance qui apparaissent sous forme de chutes de tension.

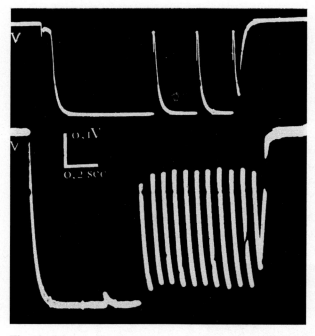

Fig. 10. Réponse d'une membrane d'huile de lin et d'huile de tung à une onde rectangulaire d'un courant constant d'une durée de 1,4 sec. *Tracé supérieur*: courant de 10^{-8} amp. La réponse rythmée selon une fréquence d'environ 5/sec survient après une latence d'environ 0,7 sec. *Tracé inférieur*: même expérience avec un courant d'intensité double. Dans ce cas la fréquence s'élève à 15/sec. La latence diminue. On notera qu'une réponse avortée survient après 0,4 sec seulement. Dans les deux cas, pendant la réponse, la conductance est multipliée de 5–10 fois. (D'après Sanchez et Reynier–Rebuffel 1969.)

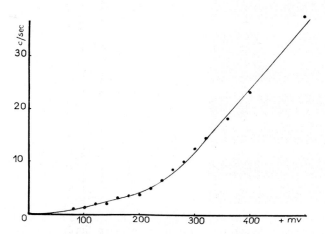

Fig. 11. Relation entre la fréquence des réponses (en réponses/sec) de la figure 10 et le voltage appliqué à la membrane.

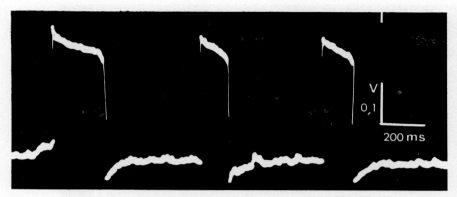

Fig. 12. Allure fréquemment observée des réponses. Les déviations vers le haut indiquent des augmentations de conductance. L'allure des réponses s'apparente à celle des électrocardiogrammes.

res dotées d'additifs appropriés. Ces phénomènes d'excitabilité s'observent même lorsque les solutions situées de part et d'autre de la membrane sont identiques, tandis que l'excitabilité de la membrane nerveuse requiert, selon Hodgkin et Huxley, une dissymétrie ionique (K^+–Na^+) de part et d'autre de celle-ci. Toutefois l'excitabilité de la membrane ne s'observe qu'en présence de solution de chlorures alcalins et non pas en présence de solutions contenant des gros cations organiques, pourtant très mobiles. Ce point sera discuté plus loin (Fig. 19).

f. *Relation intensité-durée* (Reynier-Rebuffel 1970). Si on établit brusquement un courant constant sous-liminaire à travers la membrane, la différence de potentiel s'élève et atteint graduellement un plateau. Sous un courant plus fort la différence de potentiel tend à dessiner une onde qui passe par un maximum et décroît ensuite (Fig. 13). Cette onde semble avoir la même allure que le "processus ou état d'excitation" défini autrefois (Monnier 1930, 1934). Pour un courant juste liminaire la réponse surgit au niveau du maximum de l'onde. Lorsque le courant augmente la réponse survient après une latence de plus en plus brève, ce qui représente une relation intensité-durée très analogue dans sa forme à celle observée sur un nerf (Fig. 14).

g. *Inefficacité relative des courants lentement croissants* (Reynier-Rebuffel 1970). Ce phénomène classique s'observe si l'on étudie la courbe intensité-différence de potentiel, d'une membrane d'huile de lin au moyen d'une tension ou d'un courant clampés lentement croissants. Il est préférable d'utiliser un courant clampé au lieu d'un *voltage clamp*; en effet dans ce dernier cas, lorsque survient la réponse, l'intensité du courant augmente souvent considérablement, de sorte que les propriétés de la membrane s'altèrent rapidement.

Si l'on utilise un courant clampé dont la croissance est ralentie par un système résistance-capacité, la tension liminaire pour laquelle apparaît la réponse est très supérieure à celle correspondant à l'emploi d'un courant à début brusque.

h. *Impédance des membranes d'huile de lin*. Si on introduit la membrane dans un pont de Wheatstone alimenté en courant alternatif, on constate que l'équilibre du pont ne peut être établi que par l'ajustement d'une capacité C_s et d'une résistance R_s en série insérées dans une branche du pont. Capacité et résistance varient avec la fréquen-

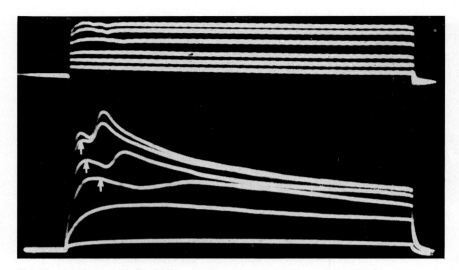

Fig. 13. Membrane d'huile de lin soumise à des passages de courant constant d'une durée de 900 msec, et d'intensité: 0,3, 0,6 ,1,0, 1,3, 1,7, 2,0 × 10⁻⁶ amp (tracés supérieurs). Ces courants déterminent les variations de potentiel (tracés inférieurs) de part et d'autre de la membrane. Au fur et à mesure que le courant s'élève, des réponses apparaissent, indiquées par des déflexions (augmentation de conductance). La latence d'apparition de ces réponses, indiquée par une flèche, diminue quand le courant s'élève.

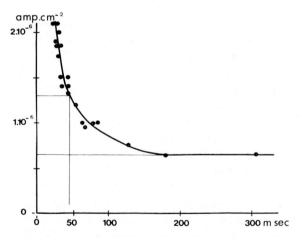

Fig. 14. Relation intensité-durée établie à partir des données de la Fig. 13. La courbe ressemble à une relation intensité-durée classique sur laquelle on peut calculer une "chronaxie" de l'ordre de 40 msec.

ce. Si on porte les capacitances $1/C_s\omega$ en ordonnées et les résistances R_s en abscisses, pour chaque fréquence de courant, on obtient un diagramme de Cole (1936) en forme de demi-cercle centré sur l'axe des abscisses (Fig. 15). Cole a démontré que ceci permet de représenter la membrane de manière formelle par une capacité C_p et une résistance R_p en parallèle. Ces paramètres sont calculables d'après le diagramme de Cole. Ils varient évidemment avec l'épaisseur de la membrane, mais en raison inverse l'un de l'autre de sorte que leur produit $R_p C_p$ (ou temps de charge) est indépendant de l'épaisseur. On voit que ce temps de charge est de quelques millisecondes, soit du même ordre que celui d'une membrane vivante.

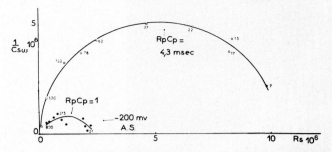

Fig. 15. Diagramme d'impédance d'une membrane d'huile de lin. *Abscisses*: résistances en série, *ordonnées*: capacitances en série utilisées pour équilibrer la membrane lorsque le pont est alimenté en courant alternatif dont la fréquence est indiquée par les chiffres portés au voisinage du cercle. Les points noirs correspondent aux mesures faites sur une membrane active soumise à une tension continue de 200 mv. Les mesures sont alors difficiles à faire, d'où leur irrégularité. Dans les deux cas le temps de charge R_pC_p est calculé. On voit qu'il diminue lors de l'activité, du fait de la diminution de la résistance R_p de la membrane.

D'une manière générale la résistance spécifique des membranes au repos se situe, lorsque d'autre part elles sont excitables, entre 1 et 10^9 ohms/cm. La constante diélectrique correspondant à la capacité C_p est comprise entre 10 et 15, c'est-à-dire intermédiaire entre la constante diélectrique de l'huile de lin originelle (2–3) et celle de l'eau qui est voisine de 80. On peut donc en déduire que le membrane excitable est une structure lipidique faiblement hydratée (Sanchez et Reynier-Rebuffel 1969).

L'impédance de la membrane lors d'une réponse est plus difficile à déterminer; il est possible toutefois d'enregistrer le déséquilibre du pont pendant une réponse (Fig. 16). Celle-ci démontre que la réponse correspond à une authentique et profonde chute de résistance. A titre de comparaison la figure classique de Cole démontrant le même phénomène au niveau de la membrane de la fibre nerveuse est reproduite.

i. *Variation d'impédance avec la température* (Fig. 17). En fonction de la température la résistance d'une membrane s'abaisse beaucoup, par exemple de 15 à 25 °C elle diminue de 3–4 fois. Cette gamme de température est d'ailleurs celle où les membranes sont les plus excitables. Au contraire, la capacité, c'est-à-dire la constante diélectrique, augmente avec la température quoique à un moindre degré, ce qui constitue une analogie de plus par rapport à la membrane de la fibre nerveuse. Mais l'augmentation de constante diélectrique avec la température constitue un paradoxe dont l'importance théorique a été récemment soulignée par Howarth *et al.* (1968). En effet la constante diélectrique de tous les corps organiques diminue avec la température, mais le phénomène inverse permet de rendre compte quantitativement du bilan des échanges thermiques très faibles qui accompagnent l'influx nerveux (Reynier-Rebuffel 1968).

Des essais récents nous conduisent à admettre qu'au cours de l'élévation de température, l'eau hydratant la membrane est de moins en moins associée à celle-ci. La quantité d'eau libre augmentant donc, il s'ensuit que la constante diélectrique de la

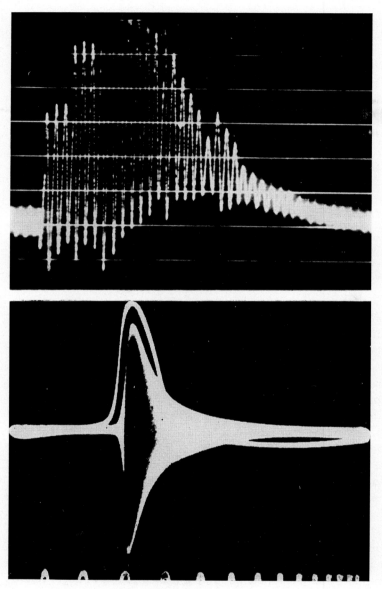

Fig. 16. *Tracé supérieur*: augmentation de conductance d'une membrane d'huile de lin au cours d'une réponse telle que celle représentée Fig. 10. La membrane est insérée dans un pont alimenté par un courant alternatif de 84 c/sec. Le pont est sensiblement équilibré entre les réponses par l'emploi d'une résistance et d'une capacité en série R_s et C_s.

Tracés inférieurs: même expérience sur la membrane d'une fibre géante de céphalopode. La courbe représente la réponse de la membrane. Celle-ci coïncide avec l'enveloppe du fuseau qui traduit le déséquilibre du pont que provoque une très forte augmentation de conductance. Fréquence du courant 10.000 c/sec. Echelles des abscisses en millisecondes. (D'après Cole 1936.)

membrane s'élève en raison de la valeur élevée de celle de l'eau (Monnier et Padrixe 1969).

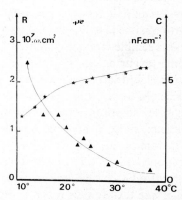

Fig. 17. Variations respectives de résistance (triangles) et de capacité (étoiles) d'une membrane en fonction de la température. La résistance diminue considérablement, tandis que la capacité augmente légèrement. Ce dernier fait se retrouve sur la fibre nerveuse.

L'excitabilité des membranes lipidiques est un phénomène très général
Les propriétés des membranes faites à partir de lipides non saturés ne dépendent pas du procédé par lequel la polymérisation oxydative de ceux-ci a été obtenue. Des réponses rythmiques d'une fréquence d'au moins 200/sec ont été observées sur une membrane résultant d'une goutte d'huile de lin étalée sur une surface d'eau pure et dont la polymérisation oxydative était effectuée à l'air sous l'action de radiations ultra-violettes (Gershfeld et Monnier, communication personnelle).

Des phénomènes d'excitabilité apparaissent aussi sur des membranes toutes diffé-rentes, par exemple sur des gels monoglycéridiques superficiels. En effet, le monooléate de glycérol (MOG) est à la fois lipophile et hydrophile. Il forme avec l'eau des gels comme l'ont montré Brokaw et Lyman (1958) et Monnier et Monnier (1968). Une cavité cylindrique en plexiglas, pourvue d'une jante creuse, est munie d'une électrode Ag-AgCl et remplie de KCl 0,1 M. Une feuille de cellophane humide est tendue sur la cavité et serrée sur la jante. Une couche mince de MOG fondu, additionné de 10% d'acide oléique est étendue au pinceau sur la feuille. En quelques minutes, la couche absorbe de l'eau à travers la feuille de cellophane et forme un gel superficiel. Une goutte de solution de KCl 0,1 M au contact avec une deuxième électrode est placée. sur le gel. La résistivité de ce dernier est en général comprise entre 1 et 5 mégΩ cm. Elle est très supérieure à celle de la feuille de cellophane humide qui ne sert que de support au gel. Lorsqu'un courant constant produit à travers le gel une différence de potentiel de 2–5 v environ, des accroissements temporaires et répétés de conductance s'observent. Ces réponses sont de même aspect que celles observées sur les membranes d'huile de lin oxydée. Toutefois, elles sont bien moins régulières et sont accompagnées d'un "bruit de fond" notable. De plus, l'ampleur de ces accroissements de conductance est moindre et ne dépasse pas 1% de la valeur de la conductance statique. La différence de potentiel pour laquelle les réponses apparaissent, est plus élevée que celle pour lesquelles l'excitabilité des membranes d'huile de lin se manifeste, sans doute en raison de la plus grande épaisseur des gels MOG (0,1–0,2 mm). L'apparition de réponses requiert l'addition préalable au MOG de 5–10% d'acide gras (acide oléique par exemple). Ceci résulte sans doute de ce que la présence de groupes anioniques est nécessaire au sein du gel et aussi parce que cette addition d'acide gras abaisse la teneur en eau du gel de 30% à environ 8%. Ce taux d'hydratation assez faible semble être une condition nécessaire à l'apparition des réponses. En effet, la même teneur en eau est atteinte et les réponses obtenues, en ajoutant 2% seulement d'acide oléique au MOG, à condition d'incorporer à ce corps environ 8% d'un triglycéride (Monnier *et al.* 1965a, b). L'uniformité et la régularité des réponses sont accrues si les solutions aqueuses adjacentes contiennent quelques millimoles de Ca^{++} ou, mieux, si 5% d'oléate de Ca^{++} est, au préalable, incorporée au MOG. L'analogie de l'action que les ions Ca^{++} exercent sur les membranes vivantes est ici évidente. Il se peut que les ions Ca^{++}, en raison de leur double charge, se comportent comme des ponts entre les charges anioniques fixées sur le gel, ce qui contribuerait à donner à ce dernier une texture plus rigide.

Enfin, les mêmes phénomènes s'observent sur des membranes formées avec d'autres dérivés lipidiques susceptibles de s'hydrater légèrement (par exemple esters phosphoriques d'alcools gras, alkyds).

En conclusion, la sélectivité ionique et l'excitabilité ne requièrent point une structure membranaire en couche bimoléculaire. Il semble donc que ces phénomènes reposent plutôt sur les caractéristiques de la membrane considérée dans sa masse. Les principales conditions requises pour l'apparition de l'excitabilité des membranes lipidiques paraissent être les suivantes: (*a*) structure semi-solide, c'est-à-dire un gel élastique formant un réseau tridimensionnel modérément hydraté. Ceci est particulièrement bien démontré par les gels de monoglycérides. Lorsque par suite d'une forte addition de triglycéride le gel ne se forme pas, aucune manifestation d'excitabilité ne s'observe; (*b*) charges ioniques fixes au sein de la membrane; (*c*) température entre 15° et 30 °C, l'optimum étant situé pour les membranes d'huile de lin et de MOG vers 21–24 °C; (*d*) pH entre 5 et 7.

Le mécanisme même de la réponse des membranes n'est pas encore élucidé. L'effet Wien de seconde espèce a été précédemment invoqué (Monnier *et al.* 1965a, b). Il suppose que, sous l'effet du champ électrique les paires d'ions formées par les charges anioniques fixées à la membrane et les cations mobiles, sont dissociées, ce qui rendrait compte de l'augmentation de conductance. Mais dans la plupart des cas, le champ paraît trop faible pour que cet effet ait une ampleur suffisante, notamment sur les membranes de MOG où l'excitabilité se manifeste pour des champs n'excédant pas 100–200 v/cm.

Une hypothèse plus séduisante invoque le rôle que joueraient des liaisons hydrogène entre des groupes OH attachés aux molécules lipidiques et les molécules d'eau. Ces liaisons contribueraient à la formation d'une structure géliforme. Les cations et les groupes OH entreraient ainsi en compétition pour la capture des molécules d'eau. Le mouvement des cations dépendrait donc de la rupture de liaisons hydrogène. Peut-être la rupture de telles liaisons au sein d'une structure modérément hydratée, s'effectuerait-elle sous l'effet d'un champ faible? Mais ceci n'expliquerait pas comment les liaisons hydrogène rompues qui seraient laissées dans le sillage d'un cation en mouve-

ment se recombineraient. Toutefois, l'importance du rôle joué par les liaisons hydrogène paraît confirmée par les observations faites sur les membranes de monoglycérides.
Ces molécules en effet contiennent deux groupes OH. Elles sont donc aptes à former
des liaisons hydrogène. De plus, l'hydratation modérée des membranes, qui semble
être nécessaire à l'apparition de leur excitabilité, suggère qu'il existe, au sein de celle-ci,
d'étroits passages sur les parois desquels sont fixés des groupes OH et des groupes
acides. Dans ces étroits passages le mouvement d'un cation dépendrait essentiellement
du nombre des molécules d'eau portées par ce dernier. Ceci s'appliquerait bien entendu
aux membranes d'huile de lin oxydée. La microphotographie électronique de celles-ci
confirme ce point de vue (Fig. 18). On peut, à titre provisoire proposer le schéma

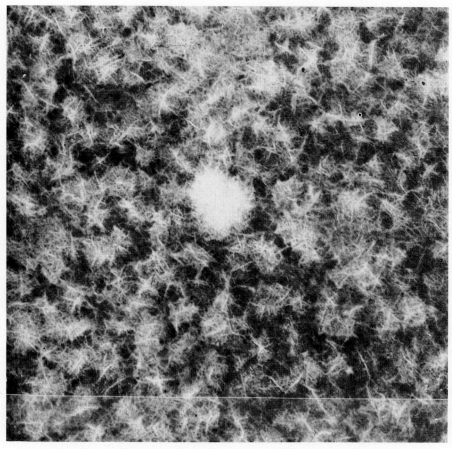

Fig. 18. Microphotographie électronique d'une membrane d'huile de lin oxydée sur MnO_4K. Les
images étoilées sont dues à la présence de microdépots de $Mn(OH)_2$ et indiquent les régions où la
polymérisation oxydative a été la plus intense. Ces étoiles paraisssent donc être l'affleurement des
fissures traversant la membrane, à la façon des fentes qui traversent un sol argileux desséché. Dans
ces fissures, sont vraisemblablement fixés des groupes acides et OH susceptibles de contracter des
liaisons hydrogène avec les molécules d'eau de la couche d'hydratation des cations inorganiques.
(Cette microphotographie est due à l'obligeance du Professeur P. Galle.) Un côte de l'image correspond à un micron.

References p. 157

suivant (Fig. 19), où est représenté un canal aqueux entouré du réticulum lipidique. Ce dernier est traversé par un pont de molécules d'eau associées par des liaisons hydrogène s'appuyant sur des groupes donneurs de telles liaisons fixés sur le réticulum. De même un cation hydraté est immobilisé par une liaison semblable. L'augmentation de conductibilité caractéristique de la réponse surviendrait quand ces liaisons hydrogène seraient rompues par le champ électrique. D'autre part, un cation organique liposoluble est figuré au sein du réticulum. Sa présence en abondance au sein de celui-ci s'expliquerait par un échange ionique résultant de l'ionisation des groupements acides fixés au réticulum. L'absence de contraintes résultant de liaisons H au sein de ce dernier rendrait compte de la grande mobilité des cations organiques dans la membrane. Des essais récents (Monnier *et al.* 1970) montrent l'importance d'un tel échange entre des lipides additionnés d'acides gras et une solution aqueuse contenant un cation organique.

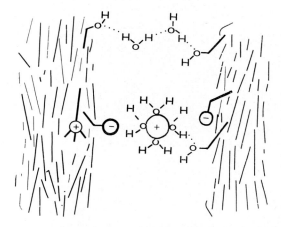

Fig. 19. Structure hypothétique d'une membrane artificielle. Un canal aqueux est entouré du réticulum lipidique. Le canal est traversé par des molécules d'eau, associées par des liaisons hydrogène, s'appuyant sur des groupes donneurs de telles liaisons fixés sur le réticulum. Un cation hydraté est immobilisé par une liaison semblable. Ces liaisons hydrogène seraient susceptibles d'être rompues par le champ électrique. Un cation organique liposoluble est figuré au sein de la membrane, sa présence en abondance au sein de celle-ci, s'expliquerait par l'ionisation des groupements acides liés au réticulum. Ce cation organique n'étant pas soumis à des liaisons hydrogène aurait ainsi une grande mobilité.

On peut se demander pourquoi il est possible de réaliser des membranes artificielles qui présentent tant d'analogies par rapport aux membranes cellulaires, en ce qui concerne la sélectivité ionique et l'excitabilité électrique. La raison du succès de tels modèles résulte sans doute de ce que, comme il est admis aujourd'hui, la réponse électrique des membranes cellulaires est en réalité un phénomène passif dont l'énergie préalable est fournie par les "transports actifs" lesquels sont mis en jeu par l'énergie résultant du métabolisme, lequel caractérise essentiellement les structures vivantes.

BIBLIOGRAPHIE

BANGHAM, A.D. *Membrane models with phospholipids: Progress in biophysics and molecular biology.* Pergamon, Oxford, **1968**, *2*: 29–95.

BROKAW, G.Y. and LYMAN, W.C. The behaviour of distilled monoglycerids in the presence of water. *J. Amer. Oil Chemists*, **1958**, *35*: 49.

COLE, K.S. and COLE, R.H. Electric impedance of Asterias eggs. *J. gen. Physiol.*, **1963**a, *19*: 609.

GOUDEAU, H. Perméabilité spécifique des membranes artificielles excitables à divers cations. *J. Physiol. (Paris)*, **1967**a, *59*: 242.

GOUDEAU, H. Perméabilité des membranes lipidiques excitables aux cations organiques et diverses drogues. *J. Physiol. (Paris)*, **1967**b, *59*: 417.

GOUDEAU, H. Caractères distinctifs du transfert des cations inorganiques et organiques au travers de membranes artificielles lipidiques. *J. Physiol. (Paris)*, **1968**, *60*: 256–257.

HOWARTH, J.V., KEYNES, R.D. and RITCHIE, J.M. The origin of the initial heat associated with a single impulse in mammalian non-myelinated nerve fibres. *J. Physiol. (Lond.)*, **1968**, *194*: 745–793.

MONNIER, A.M. Mathematical analysis applied to some functions of the nervous system. *Collecting Net (Woods Hole)*, **1930**, *5*: 178–180.

MONNIER, A.M. *L'excitation électrique des tissus.* Hermann, Paris, **1934**: 335 p.

MONNIER, A.M. et MONNIER, A. Les esters oléiques partiels du glycérol comme constituants supposés des membranes cellulaires. *J. Physiol. (Paris)*, **1958**, *50*: 416.

MONNIER, A.M. et MONNIER, A. Formation de membranes minces et stables par étalement de lipides non saturés sur des solutions oxydantes. *J. Physiol. (Paris)*, **1964**, *56*: 410.

MONNIER, A.M. et PADRIXE, J. Variation d'impédance et de structure des membranes de monogly-cérides en fonction de la température. *J. Physiol. (Paris)*, **1969**, *61*: 356.

MONNIER, A.M., GOUDEAU, H. and REYNIER-REBUFFEL, A.M. Electrically excitable artificial lipidic membranes. *J. cell. comp. Physiol.*, **1965**a, *66*: 147–154.

MONNIER, A.M., GOUDEAU, H. et REYNIER-REBUFFEL, A.M. Caractères généraux des membranes artificielles excitables. *C.R. Soc. Biol. (Paris)*, **1965**b, *165*: 252–258.

MONNIER, A.M., HOUDU, T. et PERRIN-LADREYT, C.M. Pouvoir d'échange ionique comparé des membranes et des gels lipidiques et des acides gras. *J. Physiol. (Paris)*, **1970**, *62*: 417).

MUELLER, P. and RUDIN, D.O. Action potential phenomena in experimental bimolecular lipid membranes. *Nature (Lond.)*, **1967**, *213*: 603–604.

MUELLER, P. and RUDIN. D.O. Translocators in bimolecular lipid membranes: their role in dissipative and conservative bioenergy transductions. *Currents concepts of bioenergetics.* Sanadi Ed., **1968**a: 157–249.

MUELLER, P. and RUDIN, D.O. Resting and action potentials in experimental bimolecular lipid membranes. *J. theor. Biol.*, **1968**b, *18*: 222–258.

REYNIER-REBUFFEL, A.M. Variation de la capacité des membranes lipidiques artificielles sous l'in-fluence de la température. *J. Physiol. (Paris)*, **1968**, *60*: 530–531.

REYNIER-REBUFFEL, A.M. Caractéristiques courant-tension des membranes lipidiques artificielles excitables. Sa variation en fonction du temps d'établissement du courant. *J. Physiol. (Paris)*, **1970**, *62*: 434.

SANCHEZ, V. et REYNIER-REBUFFEL, A.M. Capacité électrostatique des membranes lipidiques artifi-cielles en fonction de la fréquence du courant et des cations des phases aqueuses. *J. Physiol. (Paris)*, **1969**, *61*: 385.

SOLLNER, K. The origin of Bi-ionic potentials across membranes of high selectivity. *J. Phys. Colloid Chem.*, **1949**, *53*: 1211–1239.

Transfer Function of the Retina

OTTO D. CREUTZFELDT

Department of Neurobiology, Max Planck Institute for Biophysical Chemistry, Göttingen-Nikolausberg (W.-Germany).

This essay is dedicated to Prof. Herbert Jasper to whom this author owes much stimulation through his continuous scientific creativity and his friendship over the years. It is also a token of appreciation from my German colleagues for Dr. Jasper's many significant contributions to neurophysiological research.

The eye, like other sense organs, transforms physical energy into neuronal activity, *i.e.*, into a code which can be understood by the nervous system. A linear transformation of light intensity into neuronal spike trains would give the visual senses only little discriminative power, since light intensities under natural conditions in which visual orientation is necessary and possible for most mammalians, may vary within a range of nearly 10 log units. By various mechanisms, the eye is able to change its sensitivity according to the mean of the ambient light distribution. These mechanisms are summarized under the term "adaptation". There is now good experimental evidence that at least two different processes are involved in adaptation: (1) photochemical adaptation in the receptors themselves and (2) "neuronal adaptation" by interaction between the receptors and the neuronal elements which are centrally located from the receptors. It is assumed that the receptor output is fed into an inhibitory pool which in turn changes the gain of the receptor-bipolar transmission in proportion to the receptor output (Rushton 1965). As probable candidates for this process the connections between horizontal cells and receptors are discussed.

Weber's law: $\frac{\Delta I}{I}$ = constant, requires that the adaptation process is directly proportional to the intensity of the adaptation light. But psychophysical measurements of the threshold at different adaptation levels show significant deviations from such direct proportionality, especially in the scotopic-mesopic range (König 1889; Barlow 1957). Recent measurements of ganglion cell sensitivities at different adaptation levels confirm these psychophysical measurements by showing that the sensitivity of the cat's retinal on-center ganglion cells in the scotopic-mesopic range does not change in proportion to I but to $I^{0.68}$ so that $\frac{\Delta I}{I^{0.68}}$ = constant (Sakmann and Creutzfeldt 1969) (Fig. 1). Thus the retina becomes relatively more sensitive at increasing adaptation levels from complete darkness up to the lower photopic range.

The excitatory input from the receptors to the ganglion cells during steady state conditions at the different adaptation levels is then $\frac{I}{I^{0.68}} = I^{0.32}$, *i.e.*, about propor-

References pp. 168–169

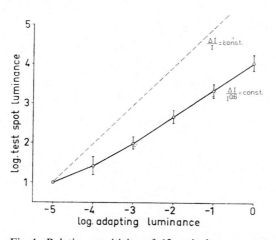

Fig. 1. Relative sensitivity of 12 retinal on-center ganglion cells at different adaptation levels. Measurements based on recordings from optic tract fibers of the cat (NO_2-anesthesia). *Ordinate*: logarithm of intensity of a test spot (diameter 20 min arc), shone into the receptive field center, which gave a criterion response of 20 spikes/sec above the maintained discharge rate during the first 250 msec after turning on the stimulus. The log values of the test spot luminance are normalized to the test spot luminance which gave a criterion response at the lowest adaptation level. *Abscissa*: logarithm of the diffuse adaptation light (I_A) in candella/m². The broken line corresponds to $\frac{\Delta I}{I}$ = const. The continuous line which connects measurements from 12 on-center ganglion cells (with standard deviation) corresponds to $\frac{\Delta I}{I_A^{0.68}}$. (From Sakmann and Creutzfeldt 1969.)

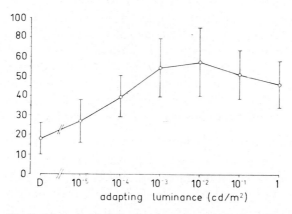

Fig. 2. Maintained discharge rate of 21 retinal on-center ganglion cells at different adaptation luminances. *Ordinate*: maintained discharge rate during the fifth minute after switching on the adaptation light. *Abscissa*: intensity of the diffuse adaptation light. D = complete darkness. Mean values from 21 on-center ganglion cells with standard deviation. Note the decrease of the mean maintained discharge rate at higher adaptation luminances. (From Sakmann and Creutzfeldt 1969.)

tional to log I. But the maintained discharge rate of retinal on-center ganglion cells does only increase at the lowest, but not at the higher adaptation levels (Fig. 2). This is due to the fact that the maintained discharge rate of a retinal ganglion cell during diffuse illumination is not the result of only the excitatory receptor-bipolar output in the receptive field center, but is the sum of the excitatory (center) and the inhibitory (surround) input (Barlow and Levick 1969; Sakmann and Creutzfeldt 1969). As a result, the signal to noise ratio increases at the higher adaptation levels and thus furthermore improves transmission through the retina. Since the relative sensitivity increase is independent of the maintained discharge rate, it can be assumed that the adaptation process takes place before the signal reaches the ganglion cell (see also Brown and Watanabe 1965; Dowling 1967; Sakmann and Creutzfeldt 1969).

The log intensity *vs.* response curves of retinal ganglion cells are S-shaped with parallel displacement at different adaptation levels (Fig. 3). At any level of adaptation

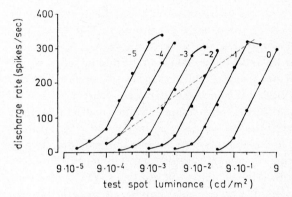

Fig. 3. Intensity *vs.* response characteristics of a retinal on-center ganglion cell at different adaptation luminances. *Ordinate*: discharge rate during the first 50 msec of the response. *Abscissa*: test spot luminance (size of test spot 20 min arc). The figures on the curves are the logarithm of the adaptation luminance at which the curves were obtained. The broken line connects responses which were obtained by stimuli of the same $\frac{\Delta I}{I}$ fraction. Note that this line is not parallel to the abscissa (which would be the case if the response were constant at identical $\frac{\Delta I}{I}$ fractions). The ganglion cell characteristics show parallel displacement and their range is less than 1.5 log unit at any adaptation level. (From Sakmann and Creutzfeldt 1969.)

they have a total dynamic range of only about 1.5 log units (Sakmann and Creutzfeldt 1969). The broken line in Fig. 3 which is drawn through points corresponding to $\frac{\Delta I}{I}$ = constant does not run parallel to the abscissa, *i.e.*, through equal response points (as would be predicted by the Weber-Fechner law), but rises with the adaptation luminance. This is in agreement with the above statement of increasing retinal sensitivity at higher adaptation levels.

The parallel displacement of the intensity *vs.* response curves indicates that the nonlinear summation (scaling) of light signals takes place at a location central to that of the adaptation process so that

$$R = a \cdot \log \frac{I}{I_A^{0.68}} = a \cdot \log I - a \cdot \log I_A^{0.68}.$$

If the adaptation process would be located centrally from the logarithmic scaling process, the slope of the log intensity *vs.* response curves should change with I_A:

$$R = a \cdot \frac{I}{I_A^{0.68}} \cdot \log I,$$

which is not the case.

Thus since neuronal (as well as chemical) adaptation take place before the signal reaches the ganglion cells and since the logarithmic scaling of light signals takes place centrally from the place of adaptation, one may ask whether the logarithmic transformation of light intensity into neuronal activity is a function of the ganglion cells themselves (Stone and Fabian 1968).

For an experimental investigation of this question we assume that the activity of many receptor-bipolar complexes converge on a single ganglion cell. The retinal area which is connected to one ganglion cell is supposed to be proportional to the extent of its dendritic tree (Brown 1965; Brown and Major 1966), and the number of receptor-bipolar ganglion cell contacts to be proportional to the density of the ganglion cell dendrites per surface area. Such a "dendritic module" explains well the sensitivity distribution across the receptive field center of a retinal ganglion cell (Creutzfeldt *et al.* 1970). With this model, we can test the two alternatives: in the case of localization of the logarithmic transformation of light intensity in the receptor-bipolar complex and of the linear summation of signals from the bipolar cells in the ganglion cell, the slopes of the log intensity *vs.* response curves of the ganglion cell responses should vary with the size of the stimulus: $R = a \cdot n \cdot \log I$, where n is the number of receptor-bipolar channels converging on the dendrites of one ganglion cell. If the ganglion cells perform the log transformation themselves, the curves should show parallel displacement proportionally to log n, since

$$R = a \cdot \log (n \cdot I) = a \cdot \log n + a \cdot \log I.$$

We have tested this with different methods (Creutzfeldt *et al.* 1970). In Fig. 4, intensity *vs.* response curves were determined with spots of light of different diameter. In the case of linear ganglion cell summation, the slopes of the curves of Fig. 4 should increase significantly with the size of the stimulus, actually in proportion to the square of the stimulus radius. This is certainly not the case. The slopes increase with the smaller diameters. With the larger diameters, the curves are displaced in parallel. The experiment has thus not clearly answered our question. Instead, the results indicate that at the small diameter and low excitation values (right side of the diagrams) the ganglion cell summation is closer to linearity (larger gain) than at large diameter and higher excitation values (left side, logarithmic scaling = smaller gain).

At this point, another aspect of the experiment of Fig. 4 should be mentioned. Apparently, the ganglion cell receives a graded input from the receptor-bipolar channels over a range of 3.5 log units, *i.e.*, from the threshold intensity of the largest stimulus (left) to the maximal response of the smallest stimulus (right). In other ganglion cells, similar ranges were found. A graded response over such a range has recently been discovered at the receptor level: Sakmann and Filion (1971) measured

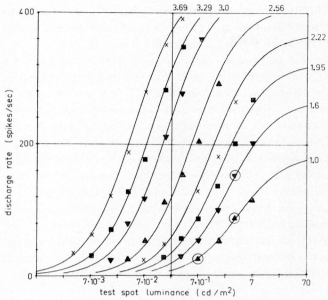

Fig. 4. Intensity *vs*. response plots of a ganglion cell obtained with stimuli of different diameter. *Ordinate*: discharge rate during the first 50 msec of the response. *Abscissa*: test spot luminance. Background illumination: 10^{-1} cd/m². The intensity *vs*. response measurements obtained at one stimulus diameter are marked by the same symbols. The logarithm of the stimulus size (retinal area illuminated by the light spot) is written beside each curve in relative values. Log I corresponds to a spot of 5 min arc diameter. The line drawn through the measurements are computer fitted curves based on equation (3), the constants a_2, b_2 and c_2 calculated from the encircled points, and on the stimulus size. Note that the slopes of the curves increase from the smallest to medium diameters, but show parallel displacement at larger diameters. The graded input into the ganglion cell ranges from the lowest point at the left ($7.10^{-3 \cdot 5}$ cd/m²) to the extreme points on the right (7 cd/m²), *i.e.* over a range of 3.5 log units. (From Creutzfeldt *et al*. 1970.)

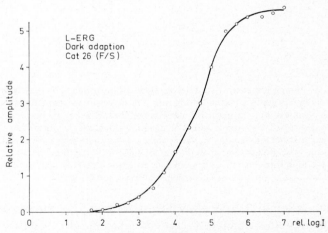

Fig. 5. Intensity *vs*. amplitude plot of the late receptor potential. The late receptor potential was measured with a micro-electrode as the local ERG about 1 week following light coagulation of the central retinal artery. The open circles represent averages of several measurements. Note the dynamic range of the graded response over 3.5 log units. (From Sakmann and Filion 1971.)

References pp. 168–169

the local receptor potential (LRP) after degeneration of the ganglion and bipolar cells following occlusion of the central retinal artery. The log intensity *vs.* amplitude plot of the LRP shows an S-shaped curve with a dynamic range of 3.5 log units (Fig. 5).

We have now the situation that the receptors transmit light intensity over 3–4 log units, and ganglion cells only over about 1.5 log units. The transfer characteristics at the two levels of the retina are S-shaped in the logarithmic plot. The lower parts of these S-shaped curves actually correspond to an almost linear summation behavior, while the flattening at the upper ends may be interpreted as a saturation phenomenon. Only the middle parts of these curves are logarithmic and can be described by R = a · log I. The situation can be represented by the diagram of Fig. 6: the thin lines are the intensity characteristics of individual receptors, the thick lines on top represent the characteristic of a retinal ganglion cell. The horizontal line is the ganglion cell threshold. If only a few receptors are stimulated by a small light stimulus, this stimulus must be bright in order to produce sufficient output from a few receptors and to reach the ganglion cell threshold. With a larger stimulus, more receptors are excited and the ganglion cell threshold is reached at lower light intensities. But in all cases, the ganglion cell shows a graded response only over the small range of its intensity characteristic.

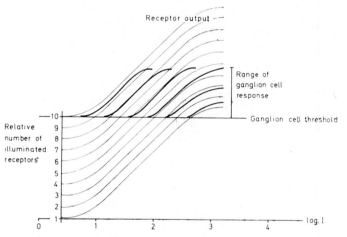

Fig. 6. Schematic representation of summation at the two different levels of the retina. The thin lines are the response characteristics of single receptors (S-shaped log intensity *vs.* response characteristics with a range of 3.5 log units). The output of each receptor-bipolar channel is represented by one characteristic: if several receptors are stimulated, the curves add. The ganglion cell sums the curves from the different receptor-bipolar channels, but its dynamic range is only 1.5 log units (thick S-shaped curves). When only "one" receptor is stimulated by a small spot of light, the ganglion threshold (horizontal line) is reached only at a high stimulus intensity, where the receptor is already near saturation. When several receptors are stimulated, the threshold is reached at lower intensities.

This experiment bears a relationship to Ricco's law which states that for a threshold response the product of intensity and stimulus size is constant (A · I = const.). Because of the linear summation of the receptors at low and the logarithmic scaling at higher intensities, Ricco's law cannot be applied to equal response experiments on single ganglion cells above threshold. In fact, the flux rates that produce equal suprathreshold responses decrease with the larger stimulus diameters (Fig. 7). At threshold, the Ricco relation should show a deviation at the largest and smallest stimuli, *i.e.*, when the light intensity is at the saturation or linear part of the receptor characteristic. In addition, the properties of the optical apparatus of the cat limits such Ricco experiments at the smaller stimulus diameters (below 5′ arc) (Wässle 1971).

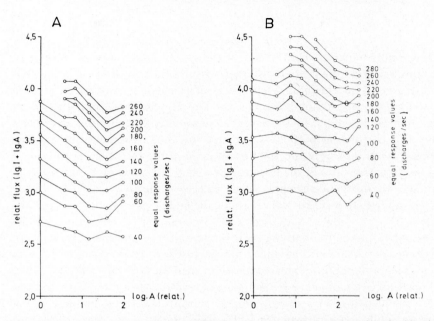

Fig. 7. Flux rate *vs.* stimulus size for different response amplitudes. The values for identical response amplitudes are connected by a line, the magnitudes of the responses (discharge rate during the first 50 msec of the response) are written beside the lines. The stimulus size (*abscissa*) is given in relative values of the stimulus area (log A), the flux (*ordinate*) as the sum of log I + log A. Note that the flux lines run nearly parallel to the abscissa at low excitation levels (response 40/sec) and become increasingly sloped at the higher response amplitudes. (From Creutzfeldt *et al.* 1970.)

Qualitatively, the summation curves of receptors and ganglion cells are comparable. They differ only quantitatively with relation to their range. Also other receptor systems have an S-shaped characteristic in the logarithmic plot. The intermediate range of such curves can be approximated by $R = \log I + c$. Over a wider range, most intensity *vs.* response curves are better approximated by power functions of the form $R = a \cdot I^x$ for $I > X > 0$. The exponent X may be different in different receptors and sensory systems. But even such power functions never sufficiently describe the full dynamic range of a receptor system. In addition, neither the log nor the power function give a simple rationale of the summation properties of sensory systems. We have therefore suggested a mathematical formalism which satisfactorily describes the intensity transfer through any sensory system, no matter whether the gain is closer to 1 or closer to logarithmic scaling. The advantage of this simple non-linear equation is that it contains terms for possible mechanisms of the observed non-linearities in such systems (Creutzfeldt *et al.* 1970; Korn and Scheich 1971).

References pp. 168–169

The S-shaped log intensity *vs.* response characteristics indicate that the gain is nearly linear at low suprathreshold intensities, that it decreases at higher intensities (logarithmic scaling) and that near the upper range, the response saturates towards a maximal value. This behavior can be described by an equation of the general form

$$R = a \cdot \frac{I}{b + c \cdot I}.$$

(1)

This equation simply indicates that the gain of the system decreases with increase of I. The constants a, b and c are characteristics of a given system such as ion permeabilities, response kinetics of chemical receptors or of transmitter substances, relative refractory period following action potentials, and may even include geometrical properties of mechanical receptors. In the eye, the constants a, b, c are time dependent (adaptation). For our present purpose we exclude this time dependency because we only considered in our measurements the first 50 msec of the response. The quotient a/c determines the upper limit of the response as well as the slope of an intensity *vs.* response curve, and also indicates up to which value of I the curves are linear. If R is plotted against log I, an S-shaped curve results, the middle part of which is approximated by $R = d + e \cdot \log I$. A change of a/b in equation (1) leads to a parallel displacement of the curve in a semi-log plot. Equation (1) in its general form is applicable to chemical reaction kinetics and it was also used in this or in similar form to describe the behavior of photoreceptors in terms of chemical flow rates (Ranke 1961), to simulate the summation of miniature end-plate potentials (Martin 1955), to describe Na^+ and K^+ conductivities in a receptor model (Zerbst *et al.* 1965) and also to describe shunting inhibition (Furman 1965; Rushton 1965). It is clear from these variable applications that the constants of equation (1) are not specific for one single mechanism underlying the non-linear transfer behavior of a system. They actually may even be a combination of more than one of such mechanisms.

As mentioned before, we have in the retina at least two non-linear summating systems, one in the receptors, the other in the ganglion cells. In order to simulate the different range of the two levels, only the constants of equation (1) must be changed. The excitatory input which reaches the ganglion cell through one receptor-bipolar channel would be

$$E = a_1 \cdot \frac{I}{b_1 + c_1 \cdot I}.$$

(2)

The ganglion cell summates the excitatory inputs E from the different channels which were excited by a light stimulus. Since these channels have a different effect on the ganglion cell because of anatomical reasons (number of synapses in contact with the ganglion cell dendrites, see above), we cannot simply multiply the number of channels. The excitation from one channel with respect to a ganglion cell must therefore be weighted with a factor g. We can then sum the different channels $g_i \cdot E_i$ and for the excitation of the ganglion cell we obtain:

$$E_{gc} = a_2 \frac{\sum\limits_{i=1}^{n} g_i \cdot E_i}{b_2 + c_2 \sum\limits_{i=1}^{n} g_i \cdot E_i}$$

a_2, b_2 and c_2 are the summation constants for the ganglion cell. These constants can be determined from the actual experiments by taking only 3 values from the curves of Fig. 4 (encircled points). With these values in equation (3), the ganglion cell responses to stimuli of a given size and intensity can be calculated. The lines drawn through the measurements of Fig. 4 are the calculated and computer-drawn curves.[1]

We can now draw a diagram of the retina and tentatively allocate the different transfer mechanisms to the different levels of the retina (Fig. 8). The interesting aspect

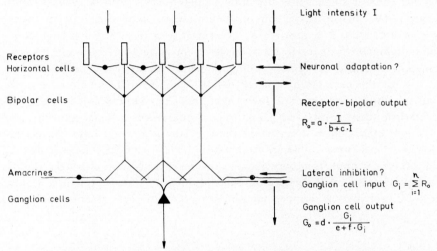

Fig. 8. Proposed model of intensity and spatial summation of retinal on-center ganglion cells.

of this model is that we do not need active inhibition within the receptive field center in order to explain the non-linear summation behavior of the retinal on-center ganglion cells as it was suggested (Rodieck and Stone 1965; Büttner and Grüsser 1968). As discussed elsewhere (Creutzfeldt et al. 1970), such a mechanism would even be incompatible with our results. One may suggest various mechanisms for the non-linear gain of the ganglion cell based on known findings of membrane physiology and synaptic transmission. In this model surround inhibition in the retina is a separate mechanism, not responsible for non-linear ganglion cell summation.

Yet we have only analyzed the summation behavior of on-center ganglion cells. The message from the retina which reaches the brain consists of on-center and off-center ganglion cell activity with almost reversed responses to retinal illumination. The data available on summation properties of off-center ganglion cells (Büttner and Grüsser 1968; Fischer and Freund 1970; Grüsser et al. 1970) indicate an identical summation behavior of retinal off-center cells.

[2] Since the dendritic density of the ganglion cells is not uniform, the actual stimulus site must be slightly corrected for the calculations (Creutzfeldt et al. 1970; Korn and Scheich 1971).

References pp. 168–169

The findings have some interesting implications for the function of the visual system. We know that at one adaptation level, the brightness distribution in our environment is approximately 1–2 log units. This corresponds well to the dynamic range of the ganglion cell. The receptor output is regulated according to a mean level of illumination by adaptation. For seeing in a dark environment, the retinal ganglion cells are able to summate activity from several receptors. This is especially the case for ganglion cells with large dendritic trees which, through bipolar cells, are in contact with many receptors (rods). This integration of activity over a relatively large area of the retina is achieved at the expense of visual acuity. At higher light intensities, this large dendritic integration field is functionally constrained by surround inhibition (Kuffler 1953; Barlow *et al.* 1957). In the fovea of primates with predominant cone vision and 1 : 1 connection between single cones and midget ganglion cells (Polyak 1944; Boycott and Dowling 1969) such a mechanism of integration of light signals from many receptors is minimal. But it is possible in the central area of cats which have good dark vision, and in both primates and cats, large receptive field ganglion cells become more prominent in parafoveal regions. Ganglion cells with large receptive fields are of limited use for the perception of small details. They probably mainly serve to perceive moving objects and objects at lower light intensities without much detail. The gain characteristic of receptors and ganglion cells guarantees a better gain at near threshold luminosities (linear summation) than at suprathreshold light intensities. There is no reason to assume a different summation behavior of the midget ganglion cells which receive an input from only one or a few receptor-bipolar channels. In this case, spatial summation can be neglected, but the intensity transfer function would follow the same principles as outlined for ganglion cells with large receptive fields.

REFERENCES

BARLOW, H.B. Increment thresholds at low intensities considered as signal/noise discriminations. *J. Physiol. (Lond.)* **1957**, *136*: 469–488.

BARLOW, H.B., FITZHUGH, R. and KUFFLER, S.W. Change of organization in the receptive fields of the cat's retina during dark adaptation. *J. Physiol. (Lond.)*, **1957**, *137*: 338–354.

BARLOW, H.B. and LEVICK, W.R. Changes in the maintained discharge with adaptation level in the cat retina, *J. Physiol. (Lond.)*, **1969**, *202*: 699–718.

BOYCOTT, B.B. and DOWLING, J.E. Organization of the primate retina: light microscopy. *Phil. Trans. Roy. Soc. Lond.*, **1969**, *B 255*: 109–176.

BROWN, J.E. Dendritic fields of retinal ganglion cells of the rat. *J. Neurophysiol.*, **1965**, *28*: 1091–1100.

BROWN, J.E. and MAJOR, D. Cat retinal ganglion cell dendritic fields. *Exp. Neurol.*, **1966**, *15*: 70–78.

BROWN, K.T. and WATANABE, K. Neural stage of adaptation between the receptors and inner nuclear layer of the monkey retina. *Science*, **1965**, *148*: 1113–1115.

BÜTTNER, U. und GRÜSSER, O.J. Quantitative Untersuchungen der räumlichen Erregungssummation im rezeptiven Feld retinaler Neurone der Katze. *Kybernetik*, **1968**, *4*: 81–94.

CREUTZFELDT, O.D., SAKMANN, B., SCHEICH, H. and KORN, A. Sensitivity distribution and spatial summation within receptive-field center of retinal on-center ganglion cells and transfer function of the retina. *J.Neurophysiol.* **1970**, *33*: 654–671.

DOWLING, J.E. The site of visual adaptation. *Science*, **1967**, *155*: 273–278.

FISCHER, B. und FREUND, H.J. Eine mathematische Formulierung für Reiz-Reaktionsbeziehungen retinaler Ganglienzellen. *Kybernetik*, **1970**, *7*: 160–166.

FURMAN, G.G. Comparison of models for subtractive and shunting lateral inhibition in receptor-neuron fields. *Kybernetik*, **1965**, *2*: 257–274.

GRÜSSER, O. J., SCHAIBLE, D. and VIERKANT-GLATKE, J. A quantitative analysis of the spatial summation of excitation within the receptive field centers of retinal neurons. *Pflügers Arch. ges. Physiol.*, **1970**, *319*: 101–121.

KÖNIG, A. Experimentelle Untersuchungen über die psychophysische Fundamentalformel in Bezug auf den Gesichtssinn. *Sitzungsber. S.-B. preuss. Akad. Wiss. Berl.*, **1889**, *27*: 641–644.

KORN, A. und SCHEICH, H. Übertragungseigenschaften der Katzenretina. *Kybernetik*, **1971**, *8*: 179–188.

KUFFLER, S. W. Discharge patterns and functional organization of mammalian retina. *J. Neurophysiol.*, **1953**, *16*: 37–68.

MARTIN, A. R. A further study of the statistical composition of the end-plate potential. *J. Physiol. (Lond.)*, **1955**, *130*: 114–122.

POLYAK, S. L. *The retina*. Chicago Univ. Press, **1944**.

RANKE, O. F. Rankes Adaptationstheorie. *Z. Biol.*, **1961**, *112*: 411–425.

RODIECK, R. W. and STONE, J. Analysis of receptive fields of cat retinal ganglion cells. *J. Neurophysiol.*, **1965**, *28*: 833–849.

RUSHTON, W. A. H. The Ferrier Lecture: Visual adaptation. *Proc. Roy. Soc. B*, **1965**, *162*: 20–46.

SAKMANN, B. and CREUTZFELDT, O. D. Scotopic and mesopic light adaptation in the cat's retina. *Pflügers Arch. ges. Physiol.*, **1969**, *313*: 168–185.

SAKMANN, B. and FILION, M. Light adaptation in the cat retina. *Vision Res.*, **1971**, *11*: 1197.

STONE, J. and FABIAN, M. Summing properties of the cat's retinal ganglion cell. *Vision Res.*, **1968**, *8*: 1023–1040.

WÄSSLE, H. Optical quality of the cat eye. *Vision Res.*, **1971**, *11*: 995–1006.

ZERBST, E., DITTBERNER, K. H. und WILLIAM, E. Über die Nachrichtenaufnahme durch biologische Receptoren. I. Theoretische Untersuchungen zur Ursache der Erregungsbildung. *Kybernetik*, **1965**, *2*: 160–168.

Specificity of Responses of Cells in the Visual Cortex

DAVID H. HUBEL

Department of Neurobiology, Harvard Medical School, Boston, Mass. (U.S.A.)

To anyone who works on the cerebral cortex, one of the most important contributions of Jasper must surely be his work with Penfield on cortical localization. It is difficult now to remember the controversies that raged a few years ago over the very existence of localization of function in the cerebrum. Perhaps the main source of doubt was the failure of experimental psychologists to demonstrate behavioural defects from cortical removals in animals such as rats. Gradually the doubts have receded, partly because more refined and imaginative behavioural methods have succeeded in showing the defects, and partly because physiologists and anatomists have amassed more and more positive evidence. An example of a behavioural defect from a brain lesion is seen in the results of corpus callosum section: this structure was thought to be useless until the experiments of Sperry and Meyers began to uncover a multitude of important and highly specific functions. The physiological results came, of course, from work such as Woolsey's on the anesthetized animal, and Penfield and Jasper's on unanesthetized man.

With many of the main areas of cortex blocked out and mapped in functional terms, the next step has been that of understanding the separate functions in detail. The somatosensory cortex receives touch and joint information from the various parts of the body surface, but what does it contribute to the analysis of those sensations? It would be preposterous to suppose that such a complex structure merely relayed the information on to still higher centers.

Considering how much is known about most organs of the body, such as the pituitary, pancreas or kidney, our slowness in coming to grips with the detailed functions of the nervous system may seem puzzling. The main source of the difficulty is to be found in the very nature of the nervous system. For most other organs it is enough, broadly speaking, to know the functions of a few classes of cells. If you understand the actions of one salivary gland cell, plus the architecture of the gland's circulation and duct system, you have a reasonable grasp of the whole organ. In the nervous system it is not enough to know how a single cell works, though of course that is essential. One must also study the connections and interrelations between enormous numbers of cells, and this is a matter of comprehending an architecture vastly more complicated than the salivary gland duct system

In the past few decades much progress has been made in working out what might be called the general cellular physiology of the nervous system, including the ionic mechanisms of impulse conduction and synaptic transmission. This has opened the way towards an attack on the functional architecture of the central nervous system. Today we are in the position of someone who has a reasonable understanding of the components of a radio circuit, the resistors, condensers, transistors and so on, but for the most part does not know how they are strung together, or what the electrical signals passing through them signify, or how the signals are being analysed or transformed.

One difficulty here is that the problem requires a study of many single cells in the intact animal. It does not get us very far to study the pooled activity of many cells at a time, for example with large electrodes placed on or in the brain, since neighbouring cells even if morphologically similar may perform entirely different tasks. Studies of populations of cells in general tell us little about the individuals. Until very recently methods for studying single cells in the intact brain did not exist and it was not until around 1950 that the first records from single cortical cells were obtained. Probably the first finding of profound interest was Mountcastle's discovery that somatosensory cells are aggregated into columnar groups according to modality. This was the first indication of a parcellation of cells into groups smaller, by an order of magnitude, than the cortical fields which the architectonic anatomists and localization neurophysiologists had fought so hard to establish in the previous decades.

In the past 10 or 15 years techniques have advanced rapidly and much progress has been made, especially in the sensory systems, where one can examine regions not too remote, in terms of numbers of synapses, from the input to the nervous system. The visual system, despite its great analytic capabilities and consequent complexity, has turned out to be especially amenable to study. This is partly because it has a fairly simple anatomic path, with flow of information directed mainly from periphery centrally over a number of relatively discrete stages. In the present paper I wish to illustrate one type of work that is being done by describing two cells in the visual cortex, one situated in area 18 in the cat, the other in area 17 in the *rhesus* monkey. These are not special or exceptional cells, but typical ones both in their specificity and their great individuality. The experiments were done at Johns Hopkins and later at Harvard by Torsten Wiesel and myself (Hubel and Wiesel 1965, 1967). In a sense they are a continuation of studies begun by Hartline in frog and *Limulus*, and by Kuffler in the cat retina.

The animal (cat or monkey) has its head firmly supported in a head holder, and the eyes are held open facing a screen 1.5 m away. Visual stimuli of various shapes, colors and rates of movement are projected upon this screen and hence onto the retinas. Records are made extracellularly from a tungsten micro-electrode introduced through a small hole in the skull. With these methods it is possible, in a good experiment, to record over 100 cells as one penetrates through 2 mm of cortex. A single cell can if necessary be studied for several hours.

Cell I: A hypercomplex cell of area 18 (visual II) in the cat
This cell was recorded from area 18, a region which, in the cat, is situated just lateral to area 17, and which receives a topographically ordered set of connections both from 17 and from the lateral geniculate body. The cell, like the great majority of cells in the visual cortex, gave no detectable response to changes in diffuse light; even shining a

bright flashlight into the eyes of the animal produced no obvious change in spontaneous firing. There were, however, strong and predictable responses to a specific stimulus within an area of visual field about 2° by 4° in size, located about 15° below and
to the contralateral side of the center of gaze. (The moon subtends 1/2° to an observer
on earth, and 1° of visual angle corresponds to about 250 μ on the cat retina.) After
much trial and error we found that the most effective stimulus was an edge, oriented in
a 2 o'clock–8 o'clock direction, with dark below and light above, swept slowly up
across the rectangular region outlined by dotted lines in Fig. 1. As the edge's position

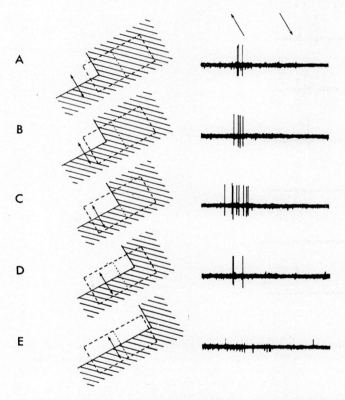

Fig. 1. Records from a hypercomplex cell in cat visual area II. Stimulation of right (ipsilateral) eye.
Receptive field, 2° × 4°, indicated by interrupted rectangle. Stimulus consisted of an edge oriented at
2 o'clock, with dark below, terminated on the right by a second edge intersecting the first at 90°.
A–C: up-and-down movement across varying amounts of the activating portion of the field; *D–E*:
movement across all of the activating portion and varying amounts of the antagonistic portion. Rate
of movement 4°/sec. Each sweep, 2 sec. (See Fig. 8 in Hubel and Wiesel 1965.)

was varied to include more and more of the left half of the rectangle, the responses
became increasingly vigorous, in terms of impulses per second and total number of
impulses (Fig. 1, *A–C*). On extending the edge still further to the right, however, the
response began to get weaker, and when it covered the entire dotted region there was no
response at all (*D–E*). It was as if stimulating the right hand area with an edge was
able to block the response that would normally have been produced by stimulating

the left area. Both regions were orientation specific. If the optimal orientation for the left region was kept constant at 2–8 o'clock, while varying the part of the edge crossing the right hand region, it was possible to show that here too a 2–8 o'clock orientation was specific, this time for a complete blocking of the response (Fig. 2).

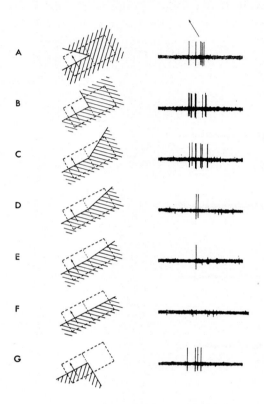

Fig. 2. Same cell as in Fig. 1. Stimulation with two intersecting edges moved up across the receptive field as shown. Inhibition is maximal when the right (antagonistic) half of the receptive fiield is stimulated with an edge having the same orientation as the optimum edge for the left (activating) half (*F*). Duration of each sweep, 2 sec. (See Fig. 9 in Hubel and Wiesel 1965.)

This cell was maximally responsive, then, to a specifically oriented moving edge terminated on the right at a specific point. If the edge extended to the right of that point the response failed, whereas it could be extended without penalty any distance to the left.

Cell II: A complex color coded cell in monkey cortex

This cell was recorded from monkey striate cortex. Like a typical cell of the type we term "complex" it gave a brisk, sustained response as a properly oriented line was swept over a restricted region of retina. Here the optimal orientation was 1 o'clock–7 o'clock; a vertical orientation or more oblique ones such as 2 o'clock–8 o'clock, or 4 o'clock–10 o'clock were quite ineffective (Fig. 3). The remarkable feature of this cell was its wave length specificity. The best responses were obtained with a moving blue line, about 480 mµ in wave-length. Wave-lengths of 520 mµ (blue green) or longer were virtually without effect, at any available brightness (Fig. 4). What was especially striking was the ineffectiveness of a *white* line, which could be obtained simply by removing the blue filter from the slide projector, *i.e.*, by adding in the longer wave-lengths that the filter had been holding back. It was as if this longer wave-length light was in some way blocking the response the blue light would have produced.

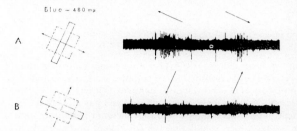

Fig. 3. Complex cell with color-coded properties recorded in layer II of monkey striate cortex. Responses to two orthogonal stimulus orientations; wave-length of light, 480 mµ (blue). Size of receptive field, $1/2° \times 1/2°$. Time for each record, 5 sec. (See Fig. 6 in Hubel and Wiesel 1967.)

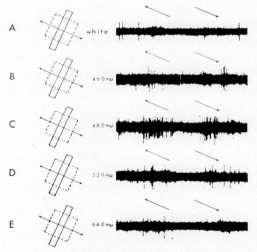

Fig. 4. Same cell as in Fig. 3. Responses to movement of optimally oriented slits of white light and monochromatic light at various wave-lengths. Monochromatic light made by interposing interference filters in a beam of white light. Stimulus energies are greatest for *A*, and progressively less for *E*, *D*, *C* and *B*. None of the responses was improved by lowering the intensity. (See Fig. 5 in Hubel and Wiesel 1967.)

DISCUSSION

My main purpose in describing these cells has been to illustrate the characteristic specificity that one finds in cells of the visual path in higher mammals. Frequently this

References p. 177

specificity seems to be the result of converging excitatory and inhibitory influences that can cancel each other. In the first example an edge crossing the left area excites, whereas an edge crossing the right area, if presented simultaneously, precisely antagonizes and cancels out this response. A plausible scheme to illustrate the mech-

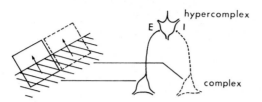

Fig. 5. Wiring diagram that might account for the properties of a hypercomplex cell. Cell responding to single stopped edge (as in Fig. 1 and 2) receives projections from two complex cells, one excitatory to the hypercomplex cell (*E*), the other inhibitory (*I*). The excitatory complex cell has its receptive field in the region indicated by the left (continuous) rectangle; the inhibitory cell has its field in the area indicated by the right (dashed) rectangle. The hypercomplex field thus includes both areas, one being the activating region, the other the antagonistic. Stimulating the left region alone results in excitation of the cell, whereas stimulating both regions together is without effect. (See Fig. 38 in Hubel and Wiesel 1965.)

anism is given in Fig. 5. It is as if the cell received an excitatory input from a cell with a receptive field in the left area, and an inhibitory input from a second cell with its field in the right hand area. A long line would be expected to fire both these lower order cells, and their influences on the cell we are discussing would cancel, resulting in no response. In the second example a similar antagonism exists between the effects of short and long wave-lengths, and we may imagine that a similar convergence of inputs is responsible for the observed behavior. The result of such transformations is that a single cell may possess specificity of response to a large number of variables, such as position on the retina, orientation, speed of movement, wave-length, line length, and so on. All of these may have to be precisely adjusted for the stimulus to work. Our impression is that for each combination of values of these variables there corresponds a cell or set of cells. Of course, this calls for a vast number of cells, but that is exactly what a structure like the visual cortex possesses, given many square centimeters of cortex, and some 10^5 cells beneath each square millimeter of surface.

By using methods such as those illustrated here to analyse a large number of cells in the visual cortex it has been possible to obtain some insight into the functions of this structure. Little by little one learns what attributes of a visual image are important in producing responses from cortical cells, and one begins to form an idea of how images are analysed. By comparing the properties of neighbouring groups of cells it is also possible to learn something of the functional architecture of the cortex, and to correlate this with morphology. At present we can thus list a number of specific functions of this part of the brain, and give definite and testable suggestions as to how these functions are carried out.

Fortunately for our livelihoods, the work is just beginning. Given the great complexity of the cortex, which is obvious from studies of its ultrastructure, it will probably be some time before any part of it is understood, except perhaps in broad outline. The encouraging thing is that it does seem possible, at least in principle, to attack the brain with present techniques, and one has the increasing confidence that it will, ultimately, be possible to understand the workings in terms of simple principles such as nerve conduction and synaptic transmission.

REFERENCES

HUBEL, D. H. and WIESEL, T. N. Receptive fields and functional architecture in two non-striate visual areas (18 and 19) of the cat. *J. Neurophysiol.*, **1965**, *28*: 229–289.
HUBEL, D. H. and WIESEL, T. N. Receptive field and functional architecture of monkey striate cortex. *J. Physiol. (Lond.)*, **1967**, *195*: 215–243.

Recent Advances and Retreats in Knowledge of Dorsal Column Function

PATRICK D. WALL

Department of Anatomy, University College, London (Great Britain)

We have been taught that dorsal columns serve Jackson's "higher centres" and "higher functions" for the somesthetic sphere. It has always been thought that destruction of this newly evolved pathway would demolish all complex perception of events on the skin leaving only crude, high threshold, poorly localized sensibilities intact. In fact the diseases which show the so called "dorsal column signs" of loss of vibration sense, two point discrimination, ability to name handled objects *etc.*, always involve structures other than dorsal columns (Petren 1902; Laidlaw *et al.* 1938; Boshes and Padberg 1953; Netsky 1953). *Tabes dorsalis*, which is the most famous, involves dorsal root destruction which cuts not only axons to dorsal columns, but also axons synapsing in dorsal horn from which run all the relayed afferent pathways. In Brown-Séquard syndrome, all ipsilateral sensory signs are attributed to dorsal column destruction in spite of the fact that we now know that important ipsilateral tracts run in the dorsolateral white matter and are also cut in this condition.

Failure to produce sensory changes by dorsal column section
The first augury of the trouble which is now upon us came when Rabiner and Browder (1948) and then Cook and Browder (1965) reported no chronic dorsal column signs in seven of the eight patients in whom they had surgically sectioned dorsal columns. The lesions extended from midline to root entry zone and were 2.5 mm deep. Fortunately for the patients, no post mortem confirmation could be obtained of the extent of the lesion and perhaps for this reason the results were neglected. In view of the highly ordered projection of dermatomes within dorsal columns, one might expect that even partial lesions of dorsal columns should produce cutaneous scotomata as predicted by Whitsel *et al.* (1970). These were not detected in these patients even, in one case, on most intensive reinvestigation (Wall 1970).

For various reasons, many teams of investigators have sectioned dorsal columns in animals who had been trained before the operation to carry out some sensory task classically attributed to dependence on impulses conducted over dorsal columns. The results have been uniformly negative in pretrained animals with histologically verified complete dorsal column sections. The following sensory tasks were tested: weight discrimination in monkeys (de Vito and Ruch 1956); conditioned forelimb flexion on touch to dogs' hind legs (Norsell 1966); tactile placing in monkey hind limbs (Christiansen 1966); cutaneous stimulus location in cats (Diamond *et al.* 1964); two point discrimination in monkeys (Levitt and Schwartzman 1966); vibration in monkeys (Schwartzman and Bogdonoff 1968); roughness discrimination in cats (Kitai and Weinberg 1968; Dobry and Casey 1970). Finally Tapper (1970), with a cat trained to respond to threshold stimuli delivered to a single tactile pad receptor, showed an improvement of performance after dorsal column section.

Is dorsal column function shared with other pathways?

Most of the authors cited explained the negative findings by postulating that dorsal columns shared a function with other projection pathways. They backed this hypothesis with the evidence that severe sensory deficits did appear if dorsal column lesions were combined with ipsilateral dorsolateral and contralateral ventral white matter lesions. However, the evolution, anatomy and physiology of the dorsal column–medial lemniscus system (DCMLS) are unique. Therefore if other tracts were capable of taking over the function of dorsal columns, they would have to do so by a different mechanism. The total size of dorsal columns has increased with respect to other tracts as mammals became more and more complex. It is hardly likely that this new system would evolve as a duplicate in case of destruction of some already extant systems. The anatomy of dorsal columns is complex and unique in at least one specific way. Certain selected peripheral axons penetrate all the way to the medulla whereas all other afferent information relays in the cord. The physiology of the DCMLS (Mountcastle 1968; Norton 1970) is also unique and highly separated from that of relayed pathways which might be carrying the same information. The special characteristics of DCMLS include high degrees of specificity and relative lack of interaction or censorship. The pathway which relays in cord with the closest similarity to DCMLS is that which runs in dorsolateral white matter from cells in lamina 4 of dorsal horn to lateral cervical nucleus and from there to thalamus. This system has been carefully studied in cat, but it is not certain that it exists in man. Some cells in the system have cutaneous receptive field sizes comparable to those in DCMLS but many different types of cutaneous afferents converge on the cells, in contrast to the strict and rigid preservation of peripheral specificity in dorsal column nuclei (Wall 1967; Brown and Franz 1969). Descending control systems markedly affect the properties of cord cells so that there is a marked difference of convergence if the cells are examined first in the decerebrate preparation and then in the spinal animal. Furthermore the properties of these cells are affected by pyramidal tract stimulation (Fetz 1968). The input–output characteristics of cord cells vary with many conditions of the freely moving animal (Wall *et al.* 1967), whereas dorsal column nucleus cells respond in a stable way (Ainsworth *et al.* 1969), except under certain specified conditions to be discussed below. We see, therefore, that the known anatomy and physiology of relayed systems does not duplicate that of DCMLS.

   If it is claimed that the relayed pathway can substitute for the new by some different mechanism, then one should be able to claim the reverse argument. Support for this view was provided by Norsell (1966) who showed that conditioned forelimb flexion to touch to hind limbs survived either dorsal column or dorsolateral fasciculus section, but was abolished by section of both. Wall (1970) tested the question directly by sectioning all white matter in thoracic cord leaving dorsal columns intact in rats. The animals appear paraplegic with lively segmental reflexes of the hind limbs, but the lumbar cord is still connected to brain by way of dorsal columns as measured histologically or physiologically by measuring conduction across the lesion region and evoked cortical potentials. In spite of the evidence that impulses were arriving over DCMLS, no hind leg stimuli could be discovered which would evoke behavioural responses in the rostral part of the animal. Stimuli rostral to the lesion produced the expected responses, but caudal to the lesion they failed to produce arousal, orientation movements, heart rate or breathing changes or an interruption of feeding. It is concluded that the functional significance of messages transmitted by DCMLS must either be to some stimulus never tested or more likely that their meaning is in relation to messages arriving over other systems. Since we must face the apparent lack of function of DCMLS in isolation and the long list of negative results, we must now turn to the few positive results of destruction to see if some testable hypothesis can be invented.

Positive findings from studies of dorsal columns
Posture. From the earliest studies, it was noticed that immediately after dorsal column section, animals left their limbs in unusual postures after completing a movement. In rats, at least, the sign disappears after some weeks. The explanation is confused by the fact that in some regions of the cord, the dorsal columns contain a special projection of primary afferents from muscle. In lower thoracic cord and lumbar regions, proprioceptive axons from hind leg are projecting to Clarke's column and, in cervical regions, axons are projecting from forelimb to external cuneate nucleus. Ferraro and Barrera (1934) and Gilman and Denny-Brown (1966) discuss the role of these special fibres and the latter authors conclude that there is a defect to be explained even when this component of dorsal columns is intact. Gaffan (1970, personal communication) has described a postural defect which long outlasts the obvious acute signs. He placed rats with unilateral dorsal column lesions on a narrow bar. He noticed that after the animal had settled down the abnormal leg tended to slip off the bar and remain extended until the animal was alerted when it returned to its normal posture.

Movement. Gilman and Denny-Brown (1966) reported that monkeys with dorsal column lesions were very unskilled in reaching out for objects, but retained great dexterity in grooming their own bodies. They also noticed that these animals retained an immobile "buddha" position in the absence of obvious disturbing stimuli. In repeating their experiment on a single monkey we have not observed the severe visuomotor deficit and one must now question the exact location of their lesions. However, Gaffan (1970, personal communication) trained rats to race down a runway from a start box to avoid shock and, in preliminary experiments, found that animals with dorsal column lesions were slower than normals.

Another quite different indication that the DCMLS is in some way involved with "voluntary movement" comes from physiological experiments. Ainsworth *et al.* (1969) noted that transmission across dorsal column nuclei, normally highly reliable, is modulated during certain phases of purposive movement. Ghez and Lenzi (1971) recorded the lemniscal response to forearm stimulation in cats during trained forearm movements and noted inhibition before and during the initiation phase of the movement.

For another type of movement, Wall (1970) reported that in rats immediately after thoracic dorsal column section, there was a diminution of head turning orientation toward a stimulus applied to the hind legs. Gaffan (1970, personal communication) in similar experiments failed to observe this deficit in chronic animals so that it may be that this defect, like the gross postural defects, is a temporary sign.

Learning. Dobry and Casey (1970) showed that extensive (67–100%) dorsal column lesions in pretrained cats failed to produce a deficit in a roughness discrimination. However two cats, with 97% and 100% of the dorsal columns destroyed, were trained after the operation and both failed to reach the criterion for discrimination grades beyond the crudest. By contrast, cats with up to 85% of their dorsal columns destroyed earned the most difficult discrimination as quickly as the controls.

l

A tentative testable hypothesis

We must try to reconcile the series of well confirmed negative findings and the disparate and often less certain positive findings. One hypothesis is that DCMLS functions as a sensory pathway where active exploration of the external world is required to provide sensory information for discriminative acts. The functional significance of these impulses is not to evoke conscious sensation or decision. Their function is rather to alert and inform central structures by way of the cortex that certain peripheral phenomena exist. This announcement is followed by decision on the part of central structures as to how sensory information arriving over relayed pathways should be handled. Descending pathways then select that sensory information from the ascending messages so that relevant information is available. This model would explain why the passive and pretrained alerted animal is able to carry out discrimination in the absence of DCMLS, since the animal has many clues about the existence, location and nature of the event to be discriminated. In the case of the animal with only DCMLS intact, the message evokes no reaction since descending controls have no ascending relayed messages on which to operate. In the circumstances where positive signs have followed DCMLS destruction it may be that the environment contained sufficient novel stimuli that their general nature could not be foreseen and therefore the animal became dependent on DCMLS and the re-programming orders which follow from it. The hypothesis proposes a subtle function which would be of great importance in increasing the sophistication of the somatosensory system. It gets away from the bankrupt attempt to assign certain sensations *per se* to DCMLS, but more important it suggests experiments to search for interaction between systems rather than experimental designs whose intention is to separate.

REFERENCES

AINSWORTH, A., GAFFAN, G.D., O'KEEFE, J. and SAMPSON, R. A technique for recording units in the medulla of the awake freely moving rat. *J. Physiol. (Lond.)*, 1969, *202*: 80–82.

Boshes, B. and Padberg, F. Studies on the cervical cord of man. The sensory pattern after interruption of the posterior columns. *Neurology (Minneap.)*, **1953**, *3*: 90–101.

Brown, A.G. and Franz, D.N. Responses of spino-cervical tract neurones to natural stimulation of identified cutaneous receptors. *Exp. Brain Res.*, **1969**, *7*: 231–249.

Christiansen, J. Neurological observations of macaques with spinal cord lesions. *Anat. Rec.*, **1966**, *154*: 330.

Cook, A.W. and Browder, E.J. Functions of posterior columns in man. *Arch. Neurol. (Chic.)*, **1965**, *12*: 72–79.

DeVito, J.L. and Ruch, T.C. Central pathways subserving weight discrimination in monkey. *Fed. Proc.*, **1956**, *15*: 152.

Diamond, I.T., Randall, W. and Springer, L. Tactual localization in cats deprived of cortical areas SI and SII and the dorsal columns. *Psychon. Sci.*, **1964**, *1*: 261–262.

Dobry, P.J.K. and Casey, K.L. Behavioural discriminative capacity and cortical unit responses in cats with dorsal column lesions. *Proc. Am. Physiol. Soc.*, **1970**.

Ferraro, A. and Barrera, S.E. Effects of experimental lesions of the posterior columns of rhesus monkeys. *Brain*, **1934**, *57*: 307–332.

Fetz, E. Pyramidal tract effects on interneurons in cat lumbar dorsal horn. *J. Neurophysiol.*, **1968**, *31*: 69–80.

Ghez, C. and Lenzi, G.L. Modulation of afferent transmission in the lemniscal system during voluntary movement in cat. *Pflügers Arch. ges. Physiol.*, **1971**, *323*: 273–278.

Gilman, S. and Denny-Brown, D. Disorders of movement and behaviour following dorsal column lesions. *Brain*. **1966**, *89*: 397–418.

Kitai, S.T. and Weinberg, J. Tactile discrimination of the DCLMS and spinocervicothalamic tract in cat. *Exp. Brain Res.*, **1968**, *6*: 234.

Laidlaw, R.W., Hamilton, M.A. and Bricker, R.M. The occurrence of dissociated disturbances of pallesthesia and kinesthesia. *Bull. neurol. Inst. N.Y.*, **1938**, *7*: 303.

Levitt, M. and Schwartzman, R. Spinal sensory tracts and two point discrimination. *Anat. Rec.*, **1966**, *154*: 377.

Mountcastle, V.B. Chapters In *"Medical physiology"*, *12th Ed*. Mosby, St. Louis, **1968**.

Netsky, M.G. Syringomyelia: a clinicopathologic study. *Arch. Neurol. Psychiat. (Chic.)*, **1953**, *70*: 741–777.

Norsell, U. The spinal afferent pathways of conditioned reflexes to cutaneous stimuli in the dog. *Exp. Brain Res.*, **1966**, *2*: 269–282.

Norton, A.C. Cutaneous sensory pathways: dorsal column-medial lemniscus system. U.C.L.A. Brain Information Service. Updated Review Project. **1970**.

Petren, K. Ein Beitrag zur Frage vom Verlaufe der Bahnen der Hautsinne im Rückenmarke. *Skand. Arch. Physiol.*, **1902**, *13*: 9–98.

Rabiner, A.M. and Browder, J. Concerning the conduction of touch and deep sensibilities through the spinal cord. *Trans. Amer. neurol. Ass.*, **1948**, *73*: 137–142.

Schwartzman, R. and Bogdonoff, M.D. Behavioural and anatomical analysis of vibration sensibility. *Exp. Neurol.*, **1968**, *20*: 43–51.

Tapper, D.N. Behavioural evaluation of the tactile pad receptor system in hairy skin of cat. *Exp. Neurol.*, **1970**, *26*: 447–459.

Wall, P.D. The laminar organisation of dorsal horn and effects of descending impulses. *J. Physiol. (Lond.)*, **1967**, *188*: 403–423.

Wall, P.D. The sensory and motor role of impulses travelling in dorsal columns towards cerebral cortex. *Brain*, **1970**, *39*: 505–524.

Wall, P.D., Freeman, J. and Major, D. Dorsal horn cells in spinal and freely moving rats. *Exp. Neurol.*, **1967**, *19*: 519–529.

Whitsel, B.L., Petrucelli, L.M., Sapiro, G. and Ha, H. Fibre sorting in the fasciculus gracilis of the squirrel monkey. *Exp. Neurol.*, **1970**, *29*: 227–242.

Recent Advances in the Study of Olfaction[1]

CARL PFAFFMANN

The Rockefeller University, New York, N.Y. 10021 (U.S.A.)

I join with the other participants in this meeting in honoring Herbert Jasper. My association dates back to the 1933–35 period when he was at Bradley Home at Brown University, just setting up his EEG laboratory. At that time I was a graduate student in the Psychology Department at Brown University and worked as a part-time assistant, soldering wires, moving equipment and generally helping in getting the new lab put together. Among other rewards of this apprenticeship was a free lunch for a hungry graduate student. But seriously, most important was the help and encouragement Herb Jasper gave me in pursuing my interests in the chemical senses which had already begun to develop at that time. Adrian and Hoagland had described the dorsal cutaneous nerve of the frog skin preparation, and had studied the effect of irritant chemicals and touch as stimuli thereof. With Herb's help, I prepared such a preparation and made some preliminary observations of the discharge in those nerves upon stimulation with saline solutions. I recall the thrill of hearing for the first time, spike-trains of impulses coming out of the audio-monitor upon stimulation. That was a thrilling moment, and was the first of many thrilling moments to come upon hearing spike discharges in many other preparations since then. Thus I can trace my friendship for and appreciation of Herbert Jasper back to my early formative graduate days, even though in subsequent research we have taken somewhat different paths.

Today in view of the time limitation I will restrict myself to olfactory chemoreception, leaving aside recent work on taste. Advances in this field have come not only from analytical physiological studies which I shall review, but also have been engendered by the increasing interest in the possibilities of olfactory communication not only in insects, but in vertebrates and especially mammals. I shall not say much about the question of the transducer process, for in spite of many studies and a wide scattering of theories, there is still little definitive knowledge on the first transducer step in olfactory stimulation. Theories attributing this to radiation or such other physical processes have not stood up very well and at the present time the majority opinion would favor some kind of a chemical process, an interaction between a molecule and a chemical acceptor or receptor site. That this process is some kind of a physicochemical process seems indicated by such effects as the importance of stereo or optical isomerism in the sensitivity and responses to the different molecules.

[1] This report was prepared with the aid of support from NIH Grant NS-08902. Research from the author's laboratory described herein was supported in part by NSF Grant GB-4198 and NIH Training Grant GM-1789.

References pp. 202–203

I. BEHAVIORAL AND ENDOCRINE EFFECTS OF ODORS

Let me begin by saying something of the relatively new and largely recently elaborated studies of behavioral and endocrinological effects caused by olfactory stimulation. These phenomena are subsumed under the heading of pheromones, from the Greek *pherein* (to carry) and *horman* (to excite, stimulate) (Karlson and Butenandt 1959), and are most dramatically demonstrated in mammals in the control of the ovulation and pregnancy processes in a series of mouse strains by Bruce, Whitten and their co-workers (see review in Whitten, 1969). Pregnancy block phenomenon in essence, as the name implies, results in block of implantation and growth of the fertilized ovum, if after copulation, the male is removed and a strange male replaced in the female cage. The strange male initiates endocrine changes which lead to pregnancy block. Estrous synchrony described by Whitten is a related effect. In this case, female mice isolated from all contact with males show a prolonged estrous cycle and some irregularity. A male brought into the colony room will induce an estrous acceleration and a synchrony of the estrus from the time of its introduction. These effects can be traced to the odor or olfactory (possibly vomeronasal) stimulation. This class of pheromone effect is know as the primer action. A second class of pheromone effect is the so-called releaser or stimulus response trigger effect. Here the presence of a biologically derived odor from a scent gland or excretion may induce the attraction or repulsion of another organism. The most well known and widespread of these effects, in many species of mammals, is attraction of the male by genital secretions, especially those of the estrous female. Experimental studies have now been made of these phenomena under more precise laboratory control than was formerly the case in field studies. Both classes have been observed in insects and have been described in some detail. In addition, insects secrete defensive agents which may ward off an attacking predator by its irritant or other noxious effect (Eisner and Meinwald 1966). Alarm substances alert other members of the colony in danger of attack.

Effects of a similar kind are now becoming more widely recognized in mammals and and it is about these that I wish to say a few words. Dr. Robert Johnston recently completed a Ph. D. thesis on olfactory communication (unpublished) in the hamster at my laboratory at the Rockefeller University. To give you some idea of the character of the stimulation and behavior of stimulus response pheromones, let me describe some of his studies. In this species there are two well defined, somewhat pigmented, specialized sebaceous glands at either flank, larger in the male than in the female. The structural integrity of this gland depends upon androgens. Following castration the gland of the male atrophies. Associated with this gland is a response called flank-marking, in which the glandular surface is rubbed vigorously against an object or surface in the environment by a curving motion of the body. The pressure against the object deposits the odor bearing substance. This response occurs both in males and females. In isolation, there is a relatively low frequency of marking in the home living cage as shown in the left-hand panel of Fig. 1. If, on the other hand, the male is allowed to enter another empty cage which had been formerly inhabited by another male, an increase in the marking rate is clearly discernible. If the animal enters the same cage

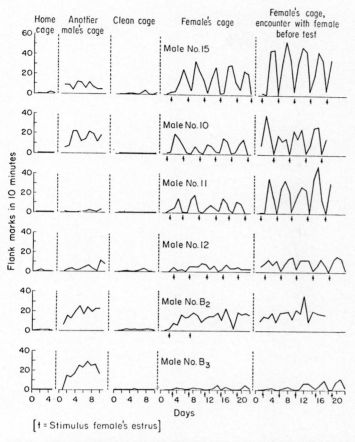

Fig. 1. Number of flank marks by males for 10 sec test intervals under different test conditions (Johnston, unpublished data).

after it has been washed, cleaned and filled with unsoiled bedding, the frequency of flank-marking is very low. When the male enters an empty cage formerly inhabited by a female, one sees an interesting cyclic pattern of flank-marking which rises to a peak between estrous periods and falls to a minimum around and just after the estrous day. The female hamster has a 4-day cycle and estrus is indicated in the figure by the arrows which clearly relate to the cyclicity in the flank-marking behavior. The graph of Male B_2 is of interest because the female ceased to show cyclic estrus after periods. Only two periods are shown, thereafter there were no cycles, and the flank-marking of the male tends to level off to a plateau, with no clear cyclicity. The strength of marking behavior may be further influenced by prior social contact among animals. The last panel shows the enhanced flank-marking following the encounter with the female prior to entering her empty cage.

Further clarification of the role of flank marking in the social behavior of the animal is given in Fig. 2 which shows flank-marking by two males before and after an encounter with each other. During the encounter the dominant animal flank-marks more

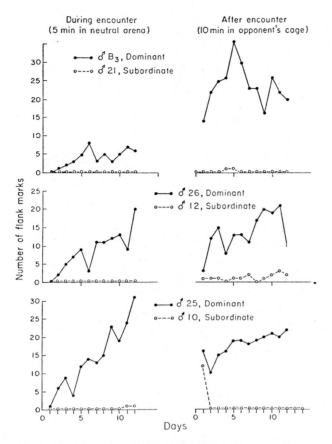

Fig. 2. Flank marks in relation to dominance in encounter between two males (Johnston, unpublished data).

frequently. During a 10-min test period after the encounter the dominant animal flank-marks a great deal but the subordinate almost not at all. Thus, Johnston concluded that flank-marking reflects aggressive motivation and dominance. This is also apparent in the non-estrous female. The females possess another source of odor from the genitalia, and they deposit the vaginal scent by lowering the genital region and pressing it against the substrate, in a dragging movement with the tail raised. It is this genital secretion which apparently accounts for the cyclicity in the males' flank-marking when introduced to the female's cage. Indeed, if the secretion is spread by an applicator upon one half of the bottom of the test cage, and the other half is left unaffected, it will be seen that flank-marking does not occur in the region with vaginal odor, but only in the half where there is no genital odor from the female. In short, the female scent attracts the male. Thus two different motivational systems appear to be instigated by these two biologically derived odors from the two different scent glands. Flank-marking is not randomly distributed throughout the test cage, but is concentrated at the spots where other animals flank-mark. The documentation on other odorous stimuli, reflecting fear, anxiety, or other motivational processes, appear to be increasing. The fascinating question of the full range of these types of odor signals, even in man, remains tantalizing, but still unanswered.

II. PHYSIOLOGY OF INSECT OLFACTION

In this section I shall review the work carried out by other workers, primarily Schneider (1969) and his colleagues, on the analysis of olfactory reception in insects where both the pheromone and non-pheromone odor reception has been carefully analyzed in recent years. Much more is known about the invertebrate case, and it provides a good model which might then be applied in part to what is currently known about vertebrate and mammalian olfactory reception. In insects the olfactory receptors are arranged in distinct units called sensilla, located mainly, but not always, on the antennae. A sensillum is typically a specialized differentiation of a cuticle, mostly of hair or peg-shaped protrusion or plate organs which consist of a large number of sensitive cells and plate-like receptor organs. The sensillum, or hair-like or peg-like structure usually has a minimum of 3 cells, 2 of which are formative, secreting the cuticle of the region, the one forming the hair, the other its socket. The third cell is a sensory neuron or primary receptor cell. The plate organs of the bee, on the other hand,

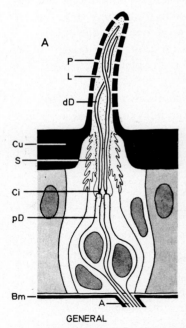

GENERAL

Fig. 3. Schematic diagram of insect olfactory sensillum in a longitudinal section. The receptor cells (white) are sheathed concentrically by the trichogen cell (light gray) and the tormogen cell (medium gray); unmodified epidermal cells are dark gray. A, axon; Bm, basal membrane; Ci, ciliary segment of dendrite; Cu, cuticle; dD and pD, distal and proximal segment of the dendrite; L, sensillar liquor; P, pore; S, dendrite sheath. (After Steinbrecht 1969.)

References pp. 202–203

have as many as 10–30 cells. Each olfactory receptor cell sends its axon (usually of very small diameter, 0.1–0.2 μ) centrally to the part of the brain that processes olfactory information. The other end of the cell, its dendrite, protrudes up from the cell body at the base into the lumen of the hair or sensillum.

Fig. 3 is a schematic drawing of a typical insect olfactory sensillum (Steinbrecht 1969). The pore-tubule system is thought to be open so that odor molecules from the outside can penetrate the cuticle and enter the fluid filled lumen of the hair containing a liquor within which the dendrites are embedded. The outermost parts of the dendrites or bundles of dendrites of the odor receptor appear to be specialized, containing only neurotubules and small vesicles, but lacking other normal cell organelles as compared with the inner dendrite.

Such olfactory sensilla are located primarily on the antennae and feelers, which vary greatly in shape. Sometimes they are short with only a few sense organs; in other cases they are thread-like and elongated as in the cockroach, shorter or densely packed as in the bee, or leaf-shaped with a feathery structure as in moths. Taste, temperature, humidity and mechanical sensitive sensilla also occur on the antennae, but the bulk of the receptors respond to odor stimulation. On the giant antenna of the male *Polyphemus* moth, there may be more than 60,000 sensilla with 150,000 receptor cells. Of these approximately 60 or 70% are specialized receptors for the sex attractant (pheromone) of the female. The antennae of the female *Polyphemus* have none of the long sensory hairs with receptors for sex odor. The female moths in the species tested do not have receptors for the sex attractants which they themselves produced although their sensory antennae contained receptors for other odors, such as food and the odor of leaves in which the eggs are laid. This dimorphism is not always the case. In the queen butterfly, both sexes respond to the sexual pheromone which is an aphrodisiac produced in the abdominal hair pencils of the male.

One of the best studied systems is that of the silkworm moth, *Bombyx mori*. The male has a large and feathery antenna which is responsive to bombykol, the sex attractant

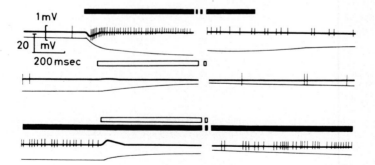

Fig. 4. Excitation and inhibition in a single olfactory unit of the carrion beetle. *Upper traces*: A.C. amplification; *lower traces*: D.C. amplification. Stimulus marked by bar above each recording. Downward deflection represents negativity of active electrode. Recordings are interrupted for several hundred milliseconds. Top record, carrion odor (filled bar): excitation. Middle record: stimulus, proprionic acid (empty bar); inhibition. Bottom record: continuous stimulation with carrion odor (filled bar, only plateau of response is shown); the additional stimulation with proprionic acid (empty bar) leads to inhibition. When proprionic acid stimulus ends, impulses return. (After Boeckh 1969.)

produced by the female moth, which is 10-trans-12-cis-hexadecadien-1-ol (Schneider 1969). The olfactory organs exhibit two types of electrical response as do other receptors. One is a slow local receptor or generator potential which originates presumably in the dendrites of the sensilla as a depolarization and the other is a series of nerve impulses which are initiated near the cell body of the receptor cell by the depolarization and travel centrally in the axons. Records from single sensilla were obtained by insterting a sharp tungsten micro-electrode needle of very small proportions near the base of an individual sensillum. This permits records of both the slow potentials and of the spike impulses initiated in that area. Fig. 4 illustrates the relation between excitation and initiation of impulses and the polarity of the response in the receptor (Boeckh 1969). With stimulus-induced negativity of the recording electrode, there is an initiation of spikes. When the polarity is reversed in the direction of hyperpolarization, there is an inhibition of activity which may have been spontaneously present. Negative potential, it is believed, reflects membrane depolarization and hence excitation; the positive potential reflects hyper- or repolarization and hence inhibition.

How is the chemical information contained in the molecules transduced and communicated to the central nervous system to initiate therein specific behavioral responses (Schneider 1969)? Research has indicated that there are two classes of olfactory cells in insects, one of which might be called "odor specialist" cells in which the response is specialized for particular pheromones, as in the case of the female attractant of the *Bombyx mori*. The *Bombyx* male reacts very strongly to the female sexual attractant, bombykol, and its geometrical isomers which were isolated and synthesized by Butenandt and Hecker (1961). The natural isomer, the trans-cis form, has the lowest threshold of the four possible isomers. Other substances, like cycloheptanone and terpineol are much weaker stimulants of these receptors, and linalool as well as some other alcohols only occasionally elicits weak reactions in the receptor. In the olfactory hairs of the *Bombyx* female the situation is quite reversed. The sexual attractant, even in exceedingly high concentrations, only induced a slight reaction in a few cases, whereas terpineol and linalool produce strong responses. It appears that the female lacks the receptors to sense its own lure substances. Most of the specialist cells when examined with a wide range of other stimulants display similar reaction spectra. In other words, they are both specific and homogeneous in their functional properties.

Specialist receptors with high specificity have also been uncovered in other species. For example, there are many thousands of odor receptors on the antennae of the male honeybee drone, some of which are specialized for the queen substance and some for the pheromone of the Nasanov gland. But in addition to these two odor specialists, the bulk of the odor receptors in the drone and worker bee seem to lack uniformity of response. There is striking variability in the action spectrum from cell to cell. This other class of olfactory receptors has been labeled "odor generalist" and in the bee and one species of moth, where up to 100 individual receptor cells were tested with a standard set of odorants, very few had similar and none had identical reaction patterns (Boeckh *et al.* 1965).

One can see, in principle, how the odor generalist would provide an ideal peripheral

References pp. 202–203

system for resolving or discriminating a large number of many different kinds of odors that might be present in the environment. To quote Schneider (1969): "Each (or a great number of them) has developed its private spectrum of reactions as a result of responding to a given compound in an excitatory or inhibitory manner, or not responding at all. The spectra of the cells do overlap considerably. It seems likely that the nerve cells of the lobe of the brain where the receptor axons terminate, or cells of higher order, could, by *knowing* the capability of each of the peripheral cells, decipher the complex odor messages from the flux of signals (plus or minus or zero) that pass to them through the fine axons of the antennal nerve". Fig. 5 illustrates a possible system

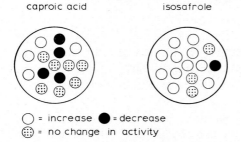

Fig. 5. Schematic representation of "generalist" response patterns across 15 olfactory neurons in olfactory nerve of honey bee to two different substances (the total number of axons is of the order of 10^5). The two different patterns across the 15 neurons could provide information for discriminating these and many other odor patterns from each other. (After Boeckh 1969.)

to permit the transmission of information of this sort. Where both generalist and specialist types can be found in one and the same organism, as in the honeybee for example, there is an obvious advantage. The specialist cells which are most numerous provide the possibility of capturing many molecules whereas the others would provide a well-graded scale for discriminating a large variety of different odor qualities (Boeckh 1969).

It is important to note that the specialist receptor system must be linked with a central neural effector system such that when the "specialist" is stimulated at much above threshold by an unnatural stimulus, the behavior ordinarily aroused by the specific hormone is also elicited. For example, the honeybee receptor specialized for the female pheromone (the queen substance) requires 10^8 molecules/cc of air; however, 10^{12} molecules of caproic acid will stimulate the receptor, seen electrophysiologically, and also lead to the behavioral response. Thus the pheromone specificity so well documented in the receptor system must be maintained in the nervous system with the appropriate brain connections for the elicitation of particular motor responses. There is thus receptor specificity and stimulus-response specificity. The mere existence of highly specific receptors for a particular pheromone at the periphery would not necessarily assure the elicitation of integrated response patterns of behavior, without an organized effector side of the system. If there were no orderly processing of the information from the specific receptors, then a high neural influx might merely arouse great chaotic neural activity. The specificity problem starts but does not end at the receptor level. We know little of the upstream neural or synaptic organization behind this

III. THE VERTEBRATE OLFACTORY SYSTEM

From insects through fishes to mammals, the receptor surfaces become progressively more buried in the nasal passages behind conchae formed by the turbinate bones. The olfactory mucosa is characterized by a yellow pigmentation, the function of which is still unknown. Supporting and sensory cells line the olfactory mucosa which is clearly distinguished from the surrounding vascular pink respiratory epithelium. Cilia of various lengths in different species project out from the sensory bipolar cells into the surrounding liquid mucus. At the outset it would appear that the invertebrate type of receptor, surrounded as it is by a hard cuticle, is very different from the protoplasmic soft structures of the vertebrate sense organ.

Steinbrecht (1969), however, has argued that the structures are basically the same and his reconstruction (Fig. 6) is drawn to show the correspondences in both. On the

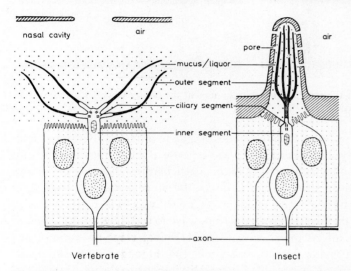

Fig. 6. Schematic comparisons between vertebrate and insect olfactory receptors to suggest analogies of structure and function (cf. Steinbrecht 1969).

left of the figure is a generalized schema of the individual cell of the vertebrate system consisting of long protruding filaments of both ciliary and outer segments, embedded in the olfactory mucus coating. The long dendritic terminations of the invertebrate receptor cells are similarly embedded in a liquor so that the molecules must be dissolved in a liquid medium before they make contact with the dendritic terminations. The air-fluid neural interface seems equivalent in both the vertebrate and the invertebrate systems. In both cases the receptor sites are presumed to be properties of the receptor cell dendritic terminations.

There is indeed a similarity in methodology in recording from the olfactory cells of an insect and the vertebrate system. It was something of a surprise to discover that spike discharges could indeed be recorded by simply driving a micropipette through the olfactory mucosa to about the level of the basement membrane (Gesteland et al.

1963). Such records utilizing both d.c. and a.c. methods show the olfactory nerve spikes superimposed upon slower receptor potentials as in the invertebrate records. Activity of single cells can be identified as trains of spikes of uniform height.

In a number of vertebrate preparations it is also possible to dissect out and record from the axons of the primary nerve cells in the olfactory mucosa as they pass to their point of entry to the brain (Shibuya and Tucker 1967). Fig. 7 illustrates the fact that

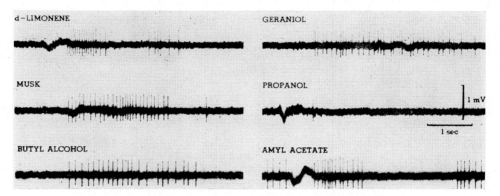

Fig. 7. Different responses of the same single olfactory unit in the turkey vulture to various odor substances (*cf*. Shibuya and Tucker 1967).

a single olfactory unit so recorded responds differentially to different olfactory stimuli with a phasic burst, steady state discharge, or no response at all, to the different substances shown. The response characteristics in this particular instance resemble those reported for the generalist receptors in the insect. In other words the individual receptors do not seem to be responsive in an "all-or-none" way to a specific stimulus or class of stimuli, rather they are differentially responsive to certain groups of stimuli. Thus, a large population of receptors with their individual response patterns for different stimuli would provide data for discriminating among a wide variety of qualitatively different odors. It is possible for the physiologist to devise a computer which could read such information. Whether the vertebrate brain indeed does so remains to be seen.

It is now evident that in all the studies that have been made at the very peripheral level, that is, by introducing micro-electrodes into the olfactory mucosa, or recording from the individual axons of the receptor cells, that the vertebrate system (including mammalian) seems to conform to the model of the insect generalist system, at least with the particular chemicals employed so far. No highly specific (sharply tuned) receptor elements in any significant numbers have yet been described even with gas chromatographically pure chemicals (O'Connell and Mozell 1969).

IV. CENTRAL PROCESSING OF OLFACTORY INFORMATION

In contrast to the insect case, the central neural connections of vertebrates and mammals, although complicated, are better understood. The ground plan of the vertebrate olfactory system is shown schematically in Fig. 8. Axons from the primary receptors enter the olfactory bulb, a kind of specialized smell brain, which lies quite anterior in the brain case. The receptor cell axons terminate in glomeruli (specialized anatomically discrete clusters or baskets of neuroterminals). Each glomerulus receives the input of about 26,000 receptors. In the rabbit 100 million primary receptors feed into 3,800 glomeruli. The glomerulus is shown in some more detail in Fig. 9. From this clustering one glomerulus has an output of only 24 large mitral cells and 68 smaller cells (Allison and Warwick 1949). The mitral cells are the origin of second order fibers which travel in the lateral and medial olfactory tracts running back to the higher brain centers. There is

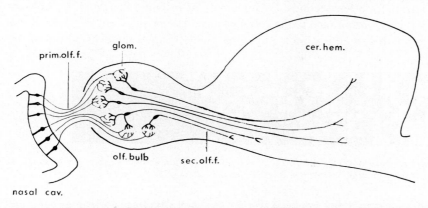

Fig. 8. Generalized schema of vertebrate olfactory system showing primary afferent cells (prim. olf. f.) leading into glomerulus and making contact with second order neurons (sec. olf. f.) (*cf.* Nieuwenhuys 1967).

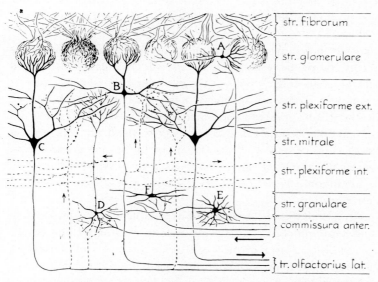

Fig. 9. Schematic drawing of neural elements in olfactory bulb including glomerulus and afferent and efferent neurons (*cf.* Lohman and Lammers 1967).

References pp. 202–203

at least 1,000–1 convergence from receptors to the second order mitral cells. It would be intriguing were each of the mitral cells to receive inputs from cells with similar functions or related characteristics. Some of the earlier experiments seemed to imply that chemically similar or qualitatively similar odors were collected together in these glomerulus clusters. Later work does not seem to bear this out.

Leveteau and MacLeod (1966 a, b) observed slow potentials from individual glomeruli using bipolar micro-electrodes, the tips of which were offset vertically by 150 μ, a distance that corresponded to the mean volume of a glomerulus. The electrical response when it occurred was taken as the response of a single glomerulus. This response appeared to be a slow monophasic potential, a few tenths of a millivolt in amplitude lasting for a few seconds. Each glomerular response appeared to be all-or-none, that is it either responded to the stimulus or remained quiescent to others. Some glomeruli responded to all 9 stimuli employed. Fig. 10 shows the distribution of the

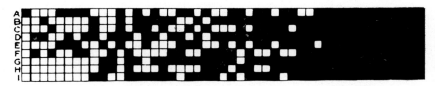

Fig. 10. Response matrix of 47 glomeruli to 9 stimuli. Histogram shows number of glomeruli responding to differing numbers of the 9 stimuli (Leveteau and MacLeod 1966a).

responses of each glomerulus (vertical column) to each stimulus (horizontal column). Black squares indicate responses, white no response. Twelve glomeruli responded to all 9 stimuli, only one glomerulus responded specifically to just one stimulus under the conditions of this experiment and only 3 pairs showed the same response spectra. All responses were excitatory, that is, depolarization and no hyperpolarization were observed.

Fig. 11, from the work of one of my former students, Donald Mathews, while we were at Brown University, shows the responsivity to different chemicals at the second order neurons beyond the glomerulus, that is at the mitral and tufted cells. At least with the chemicals employed, he did not see many highly selective units (Mathews, 1966, unpublished). Rather there appeared to be a matrix of all possible combinations of response not unlike that described for the insect generalists. In addition there was a mixture of inhibitory as well as excitatory effects in contrast to the glomerular effects. The inhibitions observed might reflect lateral interaction by way of the external plexiform collaterals. Inhibition may not occur peripherally in the vertebrate mucosa except at high concentrations.

Because most of the studies in the vertebrate and the mammalian olfactory system have employed few biological odors of possible relevance to pheromone effects, Dr. Pfaff and I in recent experiments have taken the lead from behavioral studies. Here we could identify stimuli, albeit crude ones, with important behavioral consequences.

It has been known for some time from the work of LeMagnen (1952), Carr *et al.* (1965, 1966) and others that the olfactory stimuli related to the estrous status of the

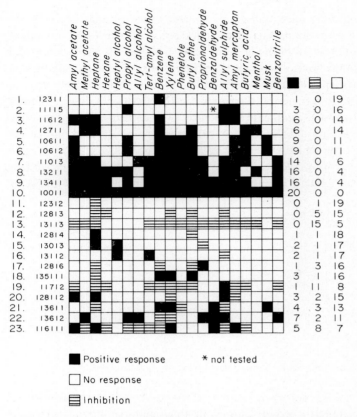

Fig. 11. Response matrix of 23 olfactory bulb units to 20 different odors in rat (Mathews, unpublished data).

female exercise a potent attraction for the male. Dr. Pfaff and I (Pfaff and Pfaffmann 1969) first confirmed that male rats, in this case Sprague-Dawley rats between 400 and 500 grams, would in fact display a behavioral preference for the odor of urine from estrous females of the same strain, in behavioral tests employed to determine the extent to which males were attracted to female urine odors.

The situation for testing responses by males to female urine odors was similar to that used by Carr *et al.* (1965). The males were tested in their home cages, the floors of which were covered with cellulose bedding. Males, housed in pairs in the home cages, were removed just before testing, and two testing glass bottles were placed in the cage. The metal screw top of each bottle had been drilled with a Teflon sleeve extended 1 inch out from the top, forming an antechamber into which the male rat could insert his nose. Each bottle contained a small amount of bedding, one clean and one soaked with 10 drops (0.5 cc) of urine from ovariectomized or estrous females.

Each test lasted 2 min and the response measure was the amount of time that the male rat extended his nose into the antechamber formed by the sleeve, *plus* the amount of time that he sniffed with his nose against the sides of the bottle *after* he had first sniffed inside the antechamber. Most of the tests were conducted "blind". On a given

References pp. 202–203

day, each male was tested only once, and all males were tested on that day with the same pair of odorants during the middle of the dark phase of a reversed day–night cycle. All males were tested on all of the odorant pairs used for 10 days. In control tests the two bottles contained only clean Sanicel bedding; one was labeled and treated as distinct. Normal, experienced males investigated containers of urine from estrous females for a significantly longer period than they did the clean containers, whereas castrated males did not show a significant difference over controls. The urine odor from nonreceptive female rats did not elicit a differential response from either the normal males or the castrated males.

We then recorded electrophysiologically from two places in the olfactory system (Fig. 12). One was in the olfactory bulb, at depths corrsponding to the mitral or

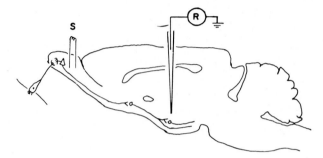

Fig. 12. Method of recording in preoptic area upon odor or olfactory bulb stimulation.

tufted cell layers. The other was somewhat more centrally in the olfactory pathways in the preoptic area and the anterior hypothalamus. In an animal like the rat there is an extensive network of fibers from the olfactory bulb and the anterior ventral cortex by way of the medial forebrain bundle. Single units were recorded with micropipettes filled with 3 M sodium chloride. Tip diameters were between 1 and 3 μ, with D.C. resistances between 0.5 and 5 MΩ. The reference electrode was clipped to the retracted skin. The micropipette was positioned by a micromanipulator according to the stereotaxic atlas of König and Klippel (1963), except for the olfactory bulb for which an atlas was not required. Electrode localization was confirmed by placing a lesion in the tissue at the tip of the pipette (50 μ amp, d.c., for 50 sec) or by marking with a dye and locating the lesion or mark in stained frozen sections. In this location we have not only moved centrally from the bulb to one of the way stations on the olfactory input, but we have examined regions with an identified relation to arousal of sexual behavior by direct neural stimulation thereof.

Conventional recording procedures were used. The frequency of spike discharges was quantitatively evaluated by use of either an integrating circuit or a spike-frequency histogram generator equipped with a Schmitt trigger and a counting circuit and write-out. Air was cleaned with silica gel and activated charcoal, and flowed past the nose of the rat at a rate measured with a flow-meter. A Sage infusion pump was used to add measured amounts of odor-saturated air from a syringe to the stream of cleaned air. In each experiment, the concentrations of all the odor stimuli were the same, between 0.01 and 0.1 saturation by volume. Urine samples for use as odor sources were collected from female rats prepared in the way described for the behavioral study. Fig. 13 illustrates the types of recording obtained from either the olfactory bulb or

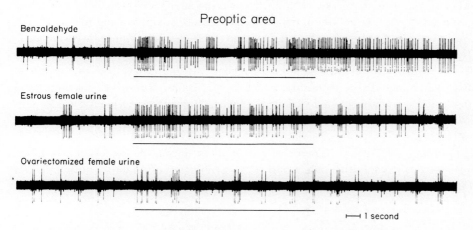

Fig. 13. Single unit activity to three stimuli from preoptic area of male rat (Pfaff and Gregory 1971).

preoptic area. The responses at both the level of the olfactory bulb (second order neurons) and in the preoptic area (third or higher order neurons) on gross inspection were very similar. That is, units responding only to one stimulus, either a chemical or a urine stimulus, were rarely observed. Many responses to odors of estrous and ovariectomized female urine were recorded from units in the olfactory bulb and preoptic area. However, no units were found which responded exclusively to either urine stimulus. Thus differential responses could indeed be observed as in prior studies with pure chemicals, but high selectivity was not immediately apparent. This perhaps may not seem remarkable since our urine stimuli were crude mixtures. But crude preparation of scent glands in *Bombyx* yielded strong antennal responses in *Bombyx* males. Other studies of crude biological material before extraction or purification have been immediately apparent in the electrophysiological chemoreceptor responses in the fish (Konishi and Zotterman 1963; Schneider 1963).

Dr. Pfaff, however, examined our data in some depth and came up with a derived measure, a differential response index which to our surprise showed that our crude urine stimuli seemed to be treated differently in the olfactory bulb and preoptic area. Responses of a neural unit to two odors were scored as differential, *i.e.*, different from each other on the basis of any one of three criteria: (a) presence *vs.* absence of a response, (b) excitation to one *vs.* inhibition to the other and (c) consistent differences in response magnitude.

The existence of a response or response-difference was determined objectively from the print out or film record as a deviation from resting activity, as compared to the variability of resting activity. In borderline cases, standard parametric statistics were used. The statistical significance of the differences between types of responses in the olfactory bulb and the preoptic area was determined by using the test for the difference between two proportions. Units that did not respond to odors were included in the statistics only when they were recorded from preparations in which at least one other unit did respond. A higher proportion of preoptic than olfactory bulb units showed differential responses to estrous *vs.* non-estrous urine odors as compared to differences among arbitrary chemical stimuli (Fig. 14). This result was promising but surprising since all the males employed in this original study were castrated. Indeed we were looking for something else when Dr. Pfaff found the differential response in the data. Drs. Pfaff and Gregory have since gone on to repeat this analysis with a new group of animals which included both normal males and castrates. Non-urine odorants were the best grades available from a variety of chemical companies. Urine for use as odorant was collected from female (200–350 gm) or male (300–400 gm) Sprague-Dawley rats as before.

Again a high proportion of preoptic area units in normal males responded differently to estrous female urine, while only a low proportion of olfactory bulb units did so (Fig. 15). The opposite was true for discrimination among non-urine odors: a higher

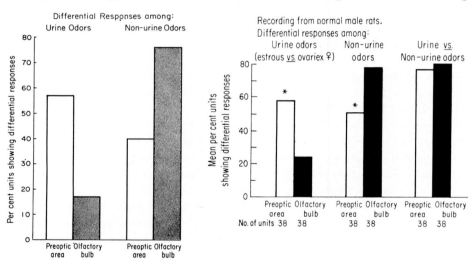

Fig. 14. Bar graph showing greater differential responses among urine odors by units in preoptic area than in olfactory bulb, compared with responses to non-urine odors (Pfaff and Pfaffmann 1969).

Fig. 15. Bar graph showing greater differential responsivity in preoptic area among urine odors than in olfactory bulb. * indicates significant differences (Pfaff and Gregory 1971).

proportion of olfactory bulb units than preoptic area units responded differentially to the members of each pair of non-urine odors. A high proportion (70–80%) of all units, both in the olfactory bulb and in the preoptic area, responded differentially when comparing urine odors to non-urine odors. The results of these differential response analyses in normal males were essentially the same as in castrated males (Pfaff and Gregory 1970).

The differential discrimination of urine *vs.* non-urine odors in the preoptic area of castrated animals, as well as normals seems paradoxical, because in behavioral preference tests the castrates are clearly different from normals: they fail to show a preference. The hormonal state of the male is not revealed in the neural discrimination mechanism in the preoptic area. In a sense this is disappointing because one might hope to find some neural mechanism where there would indeed be a correlated relation between preference behavior and physiology. If the castrated and normal animals display the same physiological differential response in the preoptic area (or elsewhere in the olfactory system), then we have not yet tapped the critical neural substrate underlying olfactory behavioral preferences.

On the other hand, finding neural responses to female urine odors in both castrated and normal animals close to the afferent input agrees with behavioral observations made earlier by Carr *et al.* (1962), namely that the presence or absence of testosterone did not seem to modify the discriminability of female estrous *vs.* non-estrous odors, as determined behaviorally. Our findings also agree with the results in another sensory domain, the genital tactile corpuscles. Cooper and Aronson (personal communication) similarly found no effect of testosterone on receptor sensitivity determined electrophysiologically. The afferent system does not appear to be tuned directly by hormonal state to receive certain information, rather it is the use that is made of that information by some upstream processing system which is dependent on hormonal state.

Let me point out, however, that our findings are to be taken as provisional pending further work, particularly with different fractions or extracts of urine of greater purity, or other genital scents or odors, or even use of other species where the behavioral responses are more sharply delineated. Furthermore, failure to find units with specific responses could be due to a number of technical difficulties in isolating such cells with the recording techniques used, to an unfortunate selection of recording sites or stimuli, poor preservation of the natural products used, or to complicating effects of anesthesia. Furthermore, I have not mentioned at all the possible involvement of the vomeronasal organ, an accessory or second olfactory type system that has a distinct neuroanatomical structure, and which feeds into the accessory olfactory bulb with a unique set of central terminations distinct from the olfactory bulb. Work on all these aspects is in progress in our laboratory.

It is also obvious that in this report, I have restricted myself to olfactory cues in signalling stimulus-response effects. Here the problem for analysis seems more direct since stimulus-response relations are immediate or relatively short term compared to the longer time scale required for primer pheromones. Some aspects of the latter have been studied with electrophysiological techniques, but not extensively. For example, Kandel (1964) demonstrated action potentials in the pituitary stalk upon electrical stimulation of the olfactory tract. More recently Scott and I (Scott and Pfaffmann 1967) have identified electrophysiologically a relatively direct olfacto–hypothalamic pathway coursing through the lateral hypothalamus *via* the median forebrain bundle in confirmation of the anatomical evidence for such connections (Powell *et al.* 1965). But Scott and Pfaff (1970) were unable to find any remarkable activity in this and other olfactory structures in the female mouse upon odor stimulation by male urine, even in females showing estrus acceleration. Their study, however, did not exhaust the subject. Relating the primer effects to olfactory physiology may well prove to be a more formidable technical problem.

References pp. 202–203

With these reservations in mind, let me review our present observations at the electro-physiological level (see also Pfaffmann 1969). We have found no evidence that bio-logically attractant sex odors, such as estrous urine, tap a uniquely sensitive receptor system in the rat. We do see evidence of selective processing of some sexually signi-ficant olfactory information upstream in the preoptic area, the region of the brain previously implicated in the modulation of sexual behavior as compared to the more peripheral parts of the olfactory system. Thus, the information already present appears to be selectively processed by way of different neural pathways, a principle that has been demonstrated in other senses, *e.g.*, in various layers of the lateral geniculate body for wave-length (*i.e.*, color), or portions of the auditory system for intra-aural time differences. The principle of selective filtering of certain stimulus features at specialized central nuclei, therefore, is not unique for the chemical senses. In future research we hope to delineate the details in olfaction and related chemical senses in this regard.

REFERENCES

ALLISON, A.C. and WARWICK, R.T.T. Quantitative observations on the olfactory system of the rabbit. *Brain*, **1949**, *72*: 186–196.

BOECKH, J., KAISSLING, K.E., and SCHNEIDER, D. Insect olfactory receptors. *Cold Springs Harbor Symposia on Quantitative Biology*, **1965**, *30*: 263–280.

BOECKH, J. Electrical activity in olfactory receptor cells. In C. PFAFFMANN (ED.), *Olfaction and Taste, III*. Rockefeller University Press, New York, **1969**: 34–51.

BUTENANDT, A. und HECKER, E. Synthese des Bombykols, des Sexuallockstoffes des Seidenspinners und seiner geometrischen Isomeren. *Angew. Chemie*, **1961**, *73*: 349–353.

CARR, W.J., LOEB, L.S. and DISSINGER, M.L. Responses of rats to sex odors. *J. comp. Physiol. Psychol.*, **1965**, *61*: 370–377.

CARR, W.J., LOEB, L.S. and WYLIE, N.R. Responses to feminine odors in normal and castrated male rats. *J. comp. Physiol. Psychol.*, **1966**, *62*: 336–338.

CARR, W.J., SOLBERG, B. and PFAFFMANN, C. The olfactory threshold for estrous female urine in nor-mal and castrated male rats. *J. comp. Physiol. Psychol.*, **1962**, *55*: 415–417.

EISNER, T. and MEINWALD, J. Defensive secretions of arthropods. *Science*, **1966**, *153*: 1341–1350.

GESTELAND, R.C., LETTVIN, J.Y., PITTS, W.H. and ROJAS, A. Odor specificities of the frog's olfactory receptors. In Y. ZOTTERMAN (ED.), *Olfaction and taste, I*. Pergamon, Oxford, **1963**: 19–34.

KANDEL, E.R. Electrical properties of hypothalamic neuroendocrine cells. *J. gen. Physiol.*, **1964**, *47*: 691–717.

KARLSON, P. and BUTENANDT, A. Pheromones (ectohormones) in insects. *Ann. Rev. Entomol.*, **1959**, *4*: 39–58.

KÖNIG, J. and KLIPPEL, R.A. *The rat brain*. William and Wilkins, Baltimore, **1963**.

KONISHI, J. and ZOTTERMAN, Y. Taste functions in fish. In Y. ZOTTERMAN (ED.), *Olfaction and taste, I*. Pergamon, Oxford, **1963**: 215–233.

LEMAGNEN, J. Les phénomènes olfactosexuels chez le rat blanc. *Arch. Sci. physiol.*, **1952**, *6*: 295–331.

LEVETEAU, J. et MACLEOD, P. La discrimination des odeurs par les glomérules olfactifs du lapin (étude électrophysiologique). *J. Physiol. (Paris)*, **1966**a, *58*: 717–729.

LEVETEAU, J. and MACLEOD, P. Olfactory discriminations in the rabbit olfactory glomerulus. *Science*, **1966**b, *153*: 175–176.

LOHMAN, A.H.M., and LAMMERS, H.J. On the structure and fibre connections of the olfactory centres in mammals. In Y. ZOTTERMAN (ED.), *Progress in brain research, Vol. 23, Sensory mechanisms*. Elsevier, Amsterdam, **1967**: 73.

NIEUWENHUYS, R. Comparative anatomy of olfactory centres and tracts. In Y. ZOTTERMAN (ED.), *Progress in brain research, Vol. 23, Sensory mechanisms*. Elsevier, Amsterdam, **1967**: 1.

O'CONNELL, R.J. and MOZELL, M.M. Quantitative stimulation of frog olfactory receptors. *J. Neuro-physiol.*, **1969**, *22*: 51–63.

PFAFF, D. and GREGORY, E. Olfactory coding in the olfactory bulb and medial forebrain bundle of normal and castrated male rats. *J. Neurophysiol.*, **1971**, *34*: 208–216.

PFAFF, D. and PFAFFMANN, C. Behavioral and electrophysiological responses of male rats to female rat urine odors. In C. PFAFFMANN (ED.), *Olfaction and taste, III*. Rockefeller University Press, New York, **1969**: 258–267.

PFAFFMANN, C. (ED.), *Olfaction and taste, III*. Rockefeller University Press, New York, **1969**: 1–648.

POWELL, T. P. S., COWAN, W. M. and RAISMAN, G. The central olfactory connexions. *J. Anat. (Lond.)*, **1965**, *99*: 791–813.

SCHNEIDER, D. Electrophysiological investigation of insect olfaction. In Y. ZOTTERMAN (ED.), *Olfaction and taste, I*. Pergamon, Oxford, **1963**: 85–103.

SCHNEIDER, D. Insect olfaction: deciphering system for chemical messages. *Science*, **1969**, *163*: 1031–1037.

SCOTT, J. W. and PFAFF, D. W. Behavioral and electrophysiological responses of female mice to male urine odors. *Physiol. behav.*, **1970**, *5*: 407–411.

SCOTT, J. W. and PFAFFMANN, C. Olfactory input to the hypothalamus: electrophysiological evidence. *Science*, **1967**, *158*: 1592–1594.

SHIBUYA, T. and TUCKER, D. Single unit responses of olfactory receptors in vultures. In T. HAYASHI (ED.), *Olfaction and taste, II*. Pergamon, Oxford, **1967**: 219–233.

STEINBRECHT, R. A. Comparative morphology of olfactory receptors. In C. PFAFFMANN (ED.), *Olfaction and taste, III*. Rockefeller University Press, New York, **1969**: 3–21.

WHITTEN, W. K. Mammalian pheromones. In C. PFAFFMANN (ED.), *Olfaction and taste, III*. Rockefeller University Press, New York, **1969**: 252–257.

Subject Index